The Power of Qi
For Health and Longevity

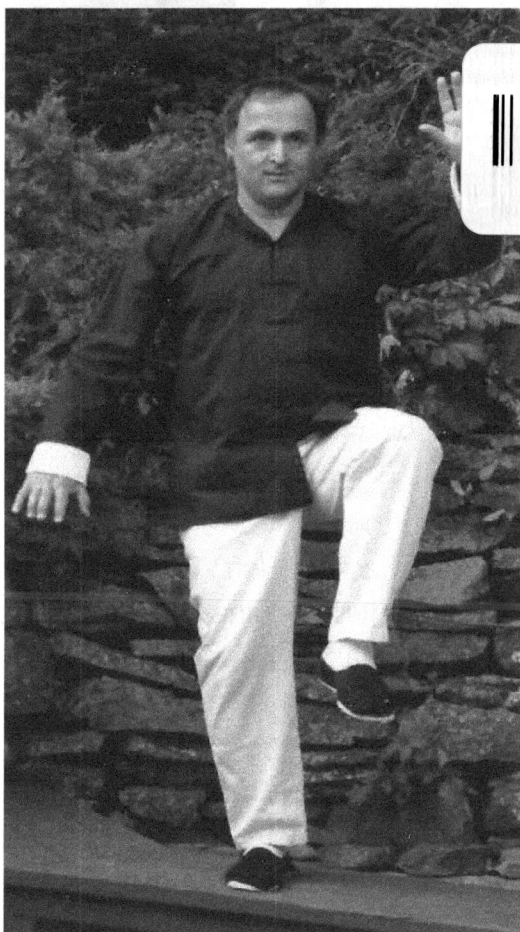

I0129779

By Maurice Lavigne, Acupuncturist
Herbalist, Qi Gong Instructor

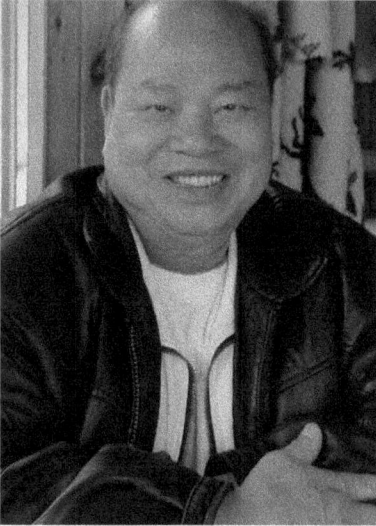
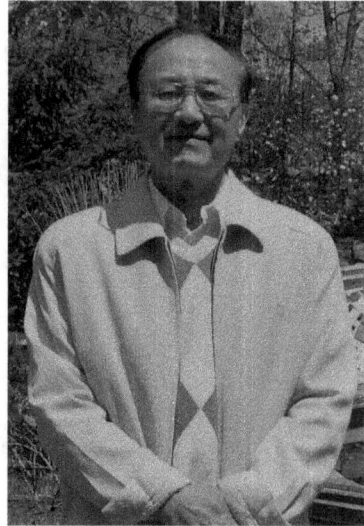

I would like to thank my two Qi Gong teachers,
Master Weizhao Wu (left) for his heart-felt
approach to Qi Gong and genuine concern for his students,
and Grand Master Tsu Kuo Shih (right)
for his generosity in sharing his vast knowledge of Qi Gong.

I have written this book to share with you the valuable
information received from my teachers over the last 20 years
and to help promote the powerful healing art of Qi Gong.

Maurice Lavigne

Table of Contents

Acknowledgements

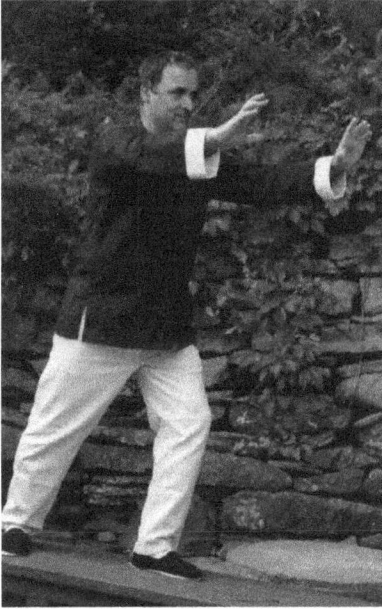

Since 1996, I have studied with three great masters of the arts of Tai Chi and Qi Gong, the late Master Weizhao Wu of Toronto, Grand Master Tsu Kuo Shih of Connecticut, USA, and Professor Huang Zhanhuan of China, founder of the Dadao style of Taijiquan.

These great masters have generously shared their passion for the arts of Tai Chi and Qi Gong. They have given their valuable time and sincere effort to help students of Tai Chi and Qi Gong better understand the true nature of these ancient martial and healing arts. For this I am very grateful. Much of the information contained in this book I have learned from them.

Many teachers have influenced my understanding of Qi. I wish to thank my first Martial Arts instructor, Wayne Thibodeau Shihan of Bathurst, New Brunswick, for introducing me to the concept of Qi, to Mahmed Benchabane of Quebec for introducing me to Ki Society Aikido, and to Massimo di Villadorata of Montreal for being my faithful Aikido teacher for 24 years.

I would also like to thank Brune Clavette of Fredericton, NB, Acupuncturist, Massage Therapist and Qi Gong Instructor, for encouraging me to become a Massage Therapist, Qi Gong practitioner and Qi Therapist.

Without the support of one's family undertaking this type of endeavor becomes very difficult if not impossible. Thank you to my business partner and wife, Louise Gosselin, and my son, Marc Antoine Gosselin-Lavigne, for supporting me in my quest to learn and teach Tai Chi and Qi Gong.

1

Preface

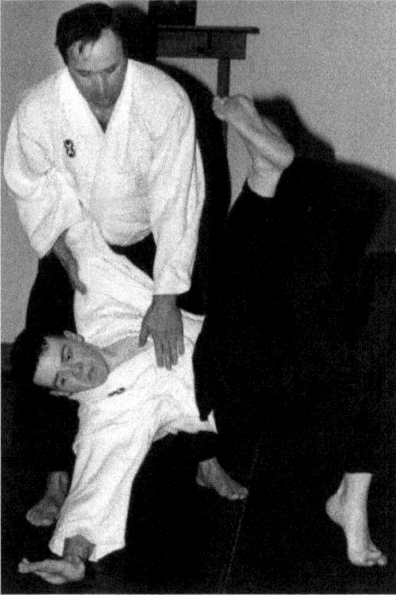

I decided to author a book on Qi Gong to share with you this immensely rich energy cultivation system. I have been studying various aspects of universal energy (Qi in Chinese – Ki in Japanese) via the martial and healing arts since 1971.

My interest in Qi dates back to my youth. I first heard about Qi in the early 70s from a local martial arts teacher, Wayne Thibodeau Shihan, who published weekly commentaries on Qi in a local community newspaper in my home town of Bathurst, New Brunswick.

In 1971, I became his student and started learning the martial art of Jui Jitsu. In those early days, there was more physical effort than Qi involved in the practice of Jui Jitsu. We spent more time with challenging workouts and powerful self-defense moves than with the study of Qi enhancing techniques.

After three years as a student of Jui Jitsu, I moved to Moncton, New Brunswick, where I studied Shotokan Karate for three years. After enrolling as a student at the local university, I discovered that one of the science teachers was offering classes in the Japanese Martial Art of Aikido.

I joined the Aikido dojo only to discover that once again there was limited instruction about Qi. Nevertheless, Aikido naturally develops a strong center or Hara, located in the lower abdomen, as well as the ability to extend one's Qi effectively via the whole body.

The objective of Aikido is the reconciliation of opposing forces in a sincere effort to resolve conflict in a peaceful manner. This self-defense art is difficult to master, as it requires an open Heart and the letting go of our innate desire to control the outcome of events.

After over 20 years of practice I obtained 3rd Dan Black Belt certification from Yoshimitsu Yamada Shihan of New York Aikikai, a direct student of the founder of Aikido, Moreihi Ueshiba. In 2013, I was promoted to the rank of 4th Dan by Osawa Hayato Shihan of Japan, Technical Director of the Canadian Aikido Federation.

In 1987 I attend a Qi Gong workshop taught by Master Yap Soon-Yeong of Malaysia. The metaphysical aspect of Master Yap's Cosmic Freedom (CFQ) Qi Gong was very intriguing, but it lacked the more physical aspects of practice I had learned to love in the martial arts.

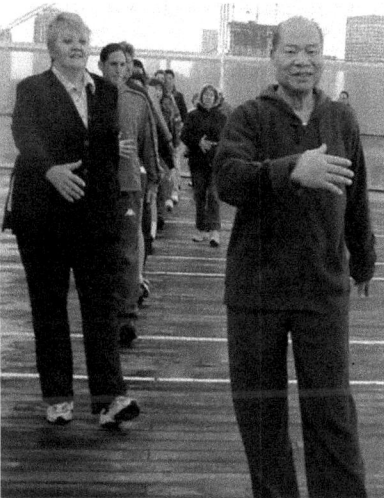

Therefore, I searched the Internet in the hopes of finding a teacher more attuned with my background. I came across a picture of a man with a big heart-felt smile and a long list of credentials. Master Weizhao Wu of Toronto, Ontario, had just emigrated from China and had opened a school of Tai Chi and Qi Gong, called Wu's Qi Gong and Tai Chi Fitness Center Inc.

I arranged for Master Wu to teach a Qi Gong workshop in Fredericton, NB. During the years that followed, as a student of Master Wu, I learned several styles of Qi Gong as well as acupressure and energy healing techniques. Master Wu can be seen in the photo teaching Walking Qi Gong during a Qi Gong workshop in Florida, USA.

While living in China, Master Wu was appointed Qi Gong Master and Liaison Man to the Chinese Qi Gong Talent Bank of the Science Research Academy, the highest official network of Chinese Qi Gong. He was also Master of four styles of Tai Chi and several styles of Kung Fu. After immigrating to Canada in the early 1990's, he created Wu's Hunyuan Gong, which he taught for over ten years in major centers across North America.

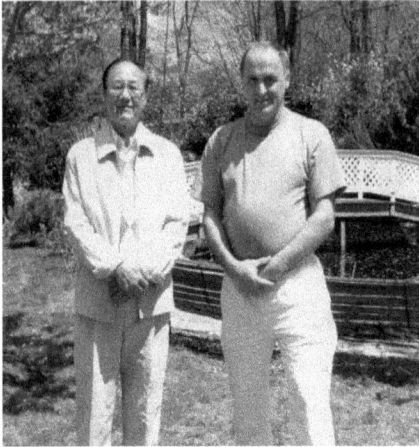

In the later years of practice with Master Wu, I started training to become a Certified Qi Healer with Qi Gong Grand Master and Doctor of Chinese Medicine, Tsu Kuo Shih, founder of the Chinese Healing Arts Center in Danbury, Connecticut, USA. In the photo, we can see Grand Master Shih and I during a Qi Gong Therapy workshop held in the summer of 2008 at the Chinese Healing Arts Center. The school, founded by Grand Master Shih, specializes in Medical Qi Gong and the training of Qi Gong therapists.

Grand Master Shih represents his family's fifth generation of Traditional Chinese Medicine Practitioners. He is a founding and honorary member of the prestigious Qi Gong Association of Beijing, and is author of numerous books and videos on Tai Chi, Qi Gong and Traditional Chinese Medicine.

Since becoming a student of Qi Gong I have received Certification in several styles of Qi Gong and Tai Chi from Master Wu as well as Certification as a Qi Healer from the Chinese Healing Arts Center.

During my years of training in Qi Gong, I enrolled in a Massage Therapy School and became a Registered Massage Therapist. I pursued my interest in Energy Healing and Acupressure Massage by studying various energy healing modalities such as Cranial Sacral Therapy, Reiki, Healing Touch, and Oriental Pressure Point Therapy.

In 2009, I was awarded a Diploma in Advanced Acupuncture from the College of Acupuncture and Therapeutics of Kitchener, Ontario, and in 2013 Certification as a Chinese Herbalist from the Institute of Chinese Herbology of Concord, California.

I practice Acupuncture, Massage Therapy, Herbology, and Qi Healing at the Fredericton Wellness Clinic Inc in Fredericton, New Brunswick, Canada, where I also teach Qi Gong classes and workshops.

Introduction

One of the fundamental concepts of Traditional Chinese Medicine (TCM) is that Qi or life energy is an invisible force that gives life to all living matter. Free flowing Qi maintains a healthy and vibrant body. A blockage in the flow of Qi eventually leads to pain and disease in the physical body.

Qi bathes the surface of every cell, forming energy currents that flow into rivers and oceans of Qi called meridians. As long as the Qi flows abundantly over each cell and in the meridians, the body is healthy.

Regular practice of Qi Gong helps to re-establish the correct flow of Qi thus improving health and longevity. Blood circulation is increased, inflammation is reduced, toxins and excess fluids are eliminated from the body. Aches and pains disappear to be replaced by a greater sense of wellness.

Acupuncture, acupressure massage, herbal formulas and natural nutrition are other methods commonly used to rebalance Qi. This book focuses mainly on the application of Qi Gong for self-healing.

Many Qi Gong styles are presented in detail including specialized forms for specific disorders such as anxiety, high and low blood pressure, and respiratory and digestive disorders.

I also offer an overview of Qi, present a view of the body's energy anatomy, and talk about how to build strong Qi through the practice of Qi Gong.

According to ancient Chinese philosophy, the condensation of wave energy into the physical world creates matter. At the end of its life cycle, matter shifts back into its original form. The Qi that moves between the physical and spiritual realms is often referred to as the Dragon.

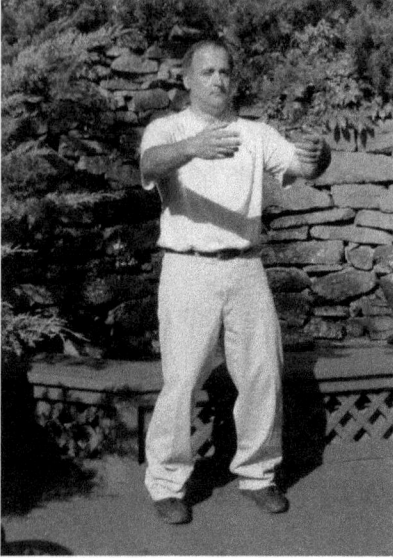

After 40 years of dedicated practice of both the Healing and the Martial arts, I have gathered together several Qi Gong styles that reflect my own personality and my understanding of the workings of Qi Gong.

From Yoga Qi Gong to the Dragon Dance, these styles help the practitioner balance the opposing and complementary forces of Yin and Yang, augmenting the flow of Qi within the body.

Students learn to clear out toxic Qi from the body, to regulate the flow of Qi, and to gather Qi from the earth, nature and the Universe. The tools used to achieve this are posture, gentle movement, stillness, breath and Mind moving Qi.

Ultimately, cultivating a compassionate heart remains at the center of all Qi Gong practice.

Secrets of Longevity

When it comes to the practice of Qi Gong it is important but sometimes difficult to find a qualified teacher. In North America, there are few standards of practice and few professional associations of Qi Gong.

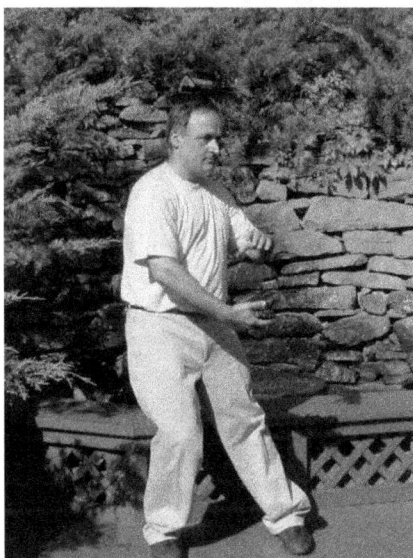

A quick search of the Internet brings up many Qi Gong styles and teachers. Some instructors have learned from schools and hospitals in China and elsewhere, others in the age-old tradition of direct transmission of knowledge from Master to student.

I have always been attracted to Qi Gong Masters who exemplify the art in their daily lives. No Master is perfect. But some live longer, happier lives than others. Their style of Qi Gong is the one I wish to learn.

What are the secrets of longevity?

According to Professor Huang Zhanhuan of China, founder of the Dadao style of Taiji Chuan, "first come down to center, calm the Mind and have no thoughts. Secondly, have a good Mind capable of love and compassion. And thirdly, cultivate life energy or Qi." According to Professor Huang, Qi Gong is the best practice for the cultivation of Qi.

In 2008, during a short visit to North America, Professor Zhanhuan gave a Tai Chi workshop where he talked about the important practice of Dan Gong. Dan refers to the Lower Dantian or energy center located in the lower abdomen. Gong means to cultivate or to nurture.

According to Professor Zhanhuan, the most important aspect of Qi Gong practice is to cultivate the essence or Jing Qi located in the Lower Dantian.

"Dan Gong is your life force. To cultivate Jing Qi do not think of anything. Feel the energy in the Lower Dantian before circulating energy elsewhere, otherwise you achieve nothing. Do not use muscular force to move the body. Use Qi. This is how to use energy properly."

Professor Zhanhuan added "walk like you are still young and keep your Spirit up. (Spirit soaring as if hung up at the Bai Hui or Crown Point by an invisible force). Accumulate Jing Qi and use it to move forward in life. This is life balance."

Ancient Masters have said that "energy gives birth to effective root and breath gives birth to Spirit. Dan Gong practice is a long-life treasure that ten thousand measures of yellow gold cannot offer."

To practice Dan Gong, rest the Mind in the Lower Dantian. This is a lot easier said than done. Keep the Mind there until the area is heavy and warm. This means you are building Jing Qi.

When you feel the energy circulating, put your Mind at the center of the circle. By regulating the breath, the Jing Qi developed with this method will foster health, wellness and longevity.

What is Qi?

"Water condenses into ice, Qi into man", Wang Chong (Ancient Sage)

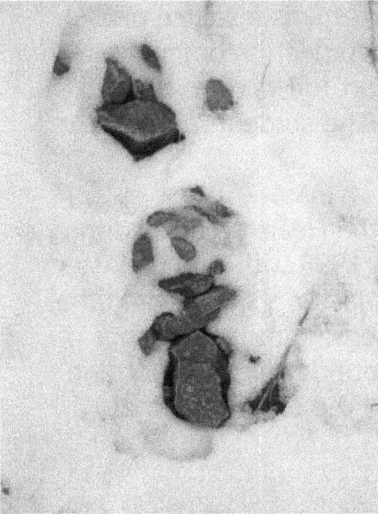

According to Traditional Chinese Medicine, Qi is the motive force behind all physiological processes. If Qi is transformed properly then birth, growth and reproduction can take place. If Qi is flourishing there is health, if it is weak or if it moves in the wrong direction there is disease. If it is balanced there is quietness.

Chinese physicians understood that everything is composed of the same energetic substance called Qi. Ancient masters concluded that although energy may appear to take on different forms, energetically everything is interconnected as one body.

According to an ancient Chinese saying, "life comes into beginning because Qi is amassed; when Qi is scattered, the person dies." Qi creates matter and acts as a medium between matter and spirit.

A famous American healer, William Gray, believed that a protective ring of energy encircles each planet and stores within it all knowledge since the beginning of time. He once said all thoughts and inventions are "taken off the ring" and anyone who listens properly can pick up whatever information he or she needs.

Gray believed the world we live in is composed of gases and energy. All substances result from unlimited combinations of energy frequencies acting on these gases. Every plant, animal and human possess their own individual energy frequency to establish and maintain life, growth and development.

Practitioners of Qi Gong can sense this energy within their own bodies and in the surrounding environment. They can also sense and sometimes see other people's energy fields. A student of Qi Gong learns not only by the spoken word but also by a transfer of energy from the instructor to the student.

Words contain energy-information. This energy is a source of knowledge that goes beyond the spoken word. It is communicated from the instructor to the student in a Heart to Heart exchange. The instructor wants to share the knowledge. The student respects the teacher and listens quietly from the Heart.

A good example of listening quietly from the Heart occurred during a teacher's Qi Gong workshop I attended in 1998 with Grand Master Shih. During the last day of class, Grand Master Shih indicated that he had a word to share with the group. Sensing the importance of the lesson, several students feverishly wrote down every word he said. We were all struggling to understand the essence of that morning's instruction.

Grand Master Shih often indicated that the palms of the hands are the antennas that capture the energy-information transmitted by the instructor. He always insisted that we place our awareness in the palms to capture his energy during lectures on Qi Gong. He explained that we must be open to the instructor to receive his or her energy and that this energy contained the information we needed to grow our Qi.

I listened both with my ears and my palms for close to three hours to no avail. Grand Master Shih was explaining a method used by teachers of Qi Gong to synchronize the energy vibrations of students in a class so that everyone would learn at the same pace.

Then suddenly out of nowhere I felt the cells of my body vibrate with those of all the other students in the room. I looked around in astonishment. At that moment, the instructor and I exchanged a heartfelt smile. He knew I had understood the nature of his teaching. I was grateful for his generosity and patience.

According to Grand Master Shih the Mind is always important in the practice of Qi Gong. With the power of the Mind we can move Qi in an instant, through objects and over vast distances. We can develop special abilities to see, to hear, to smell, to heal, and share in the power of the Universe.

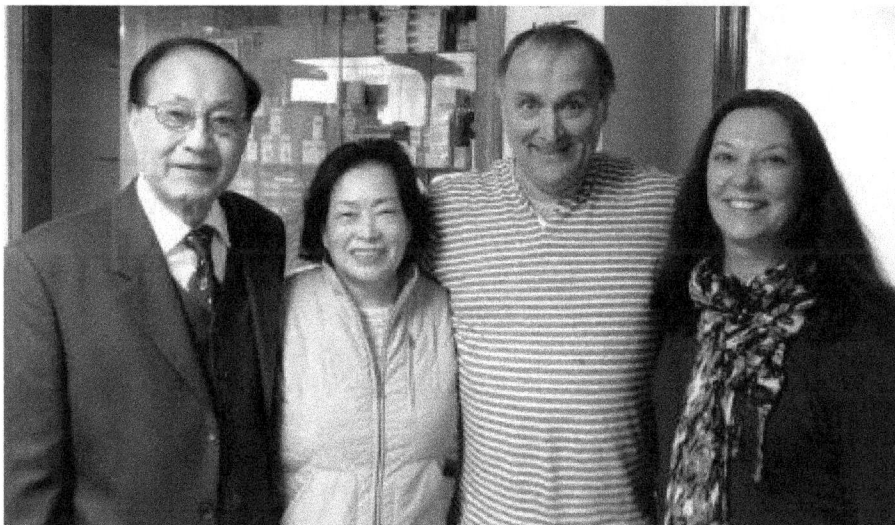

In the photo above taken in October 2014 at a Qi Healers gathering in Connecticut, USA, we can see left to right, Grand Master Tsu Kuo Shih, his wife Dr Huang, the author Maurice, with his wife, and Qi Gong practitioner and instructor, Louise.

Types of Qi

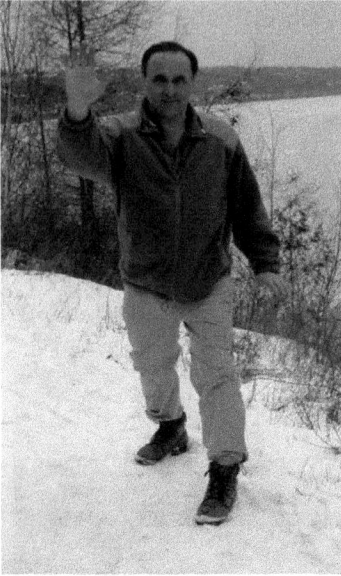

Qi can be described according to the function it fulfills in the body. I will review a few types of Qi that may be useful in the practice of Qi Gong.

- **Jing or Essence** is derived from one's parents and is supplemented by acquired Qi. It is responsible for growth, reproduction and development, is stored mainly in the Kidneys, and circulates all over the body, especially in the Eight Extraordinary Meridians.

Kidney Jing produces Marrow. The Brain in TCM is called the "Sea of Marrow". Therefore, if Kidney Jing is weak, the brain may be undernourished, leading to such symptoms as poor memory or concentration, an "empty" feeling in the head and dizziness. Weak Jing in children may lead to poor bone development, slow learning and poor concentration. Weak Jing in the elderly may lead to deafness, osteoporosis and unclear thinking.

- **Yuan Qi or Original Qi** is derived from Jing. It can be viewed as "Jing in motion". It promotes and stimulates functional activities of organs and provides the foundation or catalyst for the production of Zhen or True Qi. It originates in the Ming Men or Gate of Fire, circulates via the Three Dantians, and pools in the meridians at the Yuan Source points.

- **Kong Qi or Air Qi** originates from the air received by the Lungs.

- **Gu Qi or Essence of Food and Grain Qi** originates from the transformation of food by the Spleen in the Stomach. The Gu Qi rises to the chest where it combines with Kong Qi (Air Qi), floats down like mist from the Lungs onto the other organs below and passes to the Heart where it is transformed into Blood.

- Ying Qi or Nutritive Qi nourishes the organs and helps to produce Blood. It circulates in the main meridians in a 24-hour cycle and flows with the Blood in the main meridians and within the Blood vessels. This aspect of Qi is needled with acupuncture.

- Wei Qi or Defensive Qi helps to protect the body, warms the surface of the body and regulates body temperature by opening and closing the pores. It is found on the surface of the body and within the muscles and skin, but not within the meridians. Its circulation is dependent on the Lungs.

Qi Functions and Disharmonies

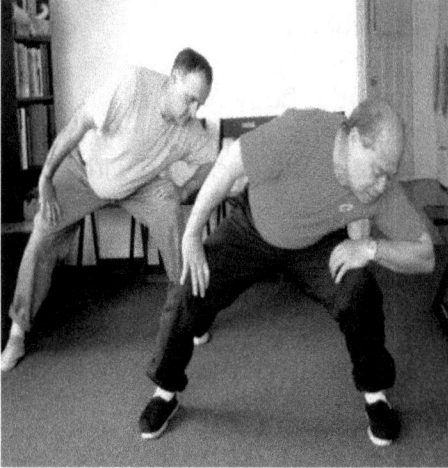

Qi supports the vital functions within the body. When a disorder arises, it is seen as a disruption in the function of Qi. A prolapsed organ, for example, is seen as a disruption in the ability of Qi to provide the raising and stabilizing function.

The formation of cysts is seen as the body's inability to adequately move Blood and manage fluids. Frequent bouts of influenza can be the result of a weakened defensive Qi, which protects the body from external pathogenic factors such as Cold and Damp.

The main functions of Qi within the body are:

- Transformation: Qi assists in the formation and transformation of fundamental substances within the body into vital energy, for example the transformation of food into Qi and Blood.

- Transportation: Qi is the foundation of all movement and growth in the body.

- Protection: Qi defends the body from external pathogens.

- Raising and Stability: Qi holds the organs in place, keeps Blood in the vessels, and governs the removal of fluids.

Whenever the movement of energy is blocked, disorders in Qi function occur. Qi has **four main states of imbalance**. These imbalances may affect many parts of the body at once or a meridian or organ system.

- Qi Deficiency: May affect the Lungs with symptoms of shortness of breath, or the Stomach and Spleen with poor appetite, fatigue and weakness. The primary treatment needed to rectify a Qi Deficiency condition is to tonify the Qi.

- Qi Stagnation: May affect the Liver and lead to chest or hypochondriac pain that is not fixed in location. The primary treatment needed to rectify Qi Stagnation is to move or regulate the Qi.

- Sinking Qi: Sinking Qi may affect the Spleen and lead to digestive issues and prolapsed organs. The primary treatment needed to rectify Sinking Qi is to raise and tonify the Qi.

- Rebellious Qi: May affect the Lungs or Stomach and lead to coughing, belching, vomiting, hiccups or dizziness. The primary treatment needed to rectify Rebellious Qi is to calm and subdue the Qi.

What is Qi Gong?

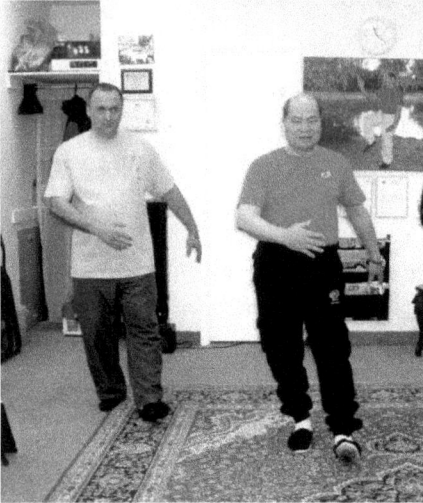

The ancient peoples of China believed that lengthening their breaths could extend their lives. This system of exercises consisted of stilling the body and the Mind, regulating breath, becoming sensitized to the movements of Qi, and finally bringing the Qi within the control of the conscious Mind.

According to A Brief History of Qi written by Zhang Yu Huan and Ken Rose, the oldest coherent system of exercises designed to guide and cultivate Qi comes from Daoist philosophers of the Warring States period (475 B.C.E. - 221 B.C.E.) of China.

In the Daoist classic of Zhuang Zi entitled Kè Yi, there are clear references to this early method of developing the power of Qi and harnessing its life extending potentials.

Qi Gong (chee-GONG) is the current name of this system of exercises. Qi means energy, the energy of the Universe. Gong means to gather with skill, thus Qi Gong is to gather energy from the Universe with practiced skill. The term Qi Gong first appeared in the book *Smart Swordsman* by Xu Xun during the Jin Dynasty.

The term Qi Gong became widely used in China in the 1950's. It referred to Qi related practices such as tranquil sitting, controlled breathing, the directing and guiding of Qi as well as the cultivation of one's moral nature to achieve a measure of skill.

There are over 3,000 forms of Qi Gong. The three major schools are medical, martial and spiritual. This book focuses mainly on the medical applications of Qi Gong.

Medical Qi Gong uses posture, gentle, slow, rhythmic movement, breath and mental imagery to clear out stagnant Qi and gather universal Qi into the body. The results of this practice are a calm Mind, energized body and a greater sense of balance, both mental and physical.

Qi Gong improves the quality of people's lives as it provides the energy to increase the body's adaptability to its surroundings, to strengthen the immune system, and to speed recovery from diseases and injury.

Why Practice Qi Gong?

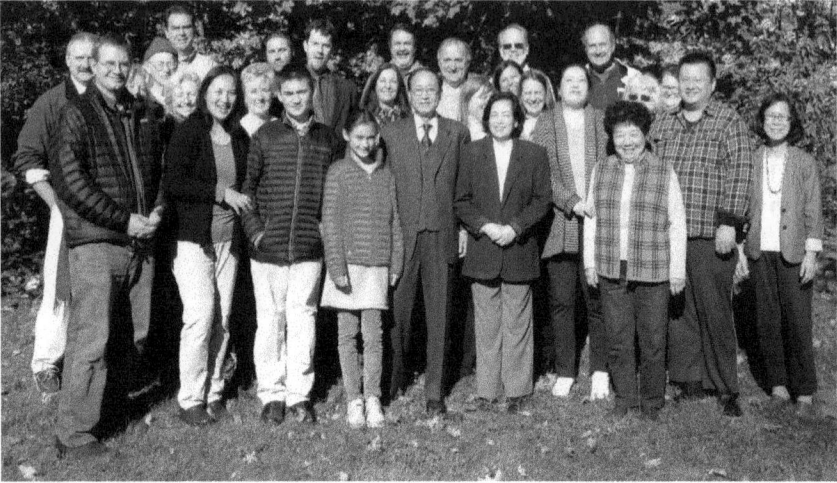

The picture shows students and family of Grand Master Tsu Kuo Shih in October 2014 during his 84th birthday celebration.

There are many reasons to practice Qi Gong. When we are weak, we build up blockages in the body's meridians or energy pathways, which impede the flow of Blood and Qi. Practicing Qi Gong helps to clear these blockages.

By concentrating on breathing, meditation, and soft movement, Qi Gong brings the body back into balance, in harmony with nature's universal rhythm. The Qi Gong student learns to build more Qi, release stagnant Qi, and direct its flow so that it spreads evenly throughout the body.

Getting enough physical exercise and following a healthy diet help increase the flow of Qi. We can also grow our Qi with specific Qi cultivation exercises.

Regular practice of Qi Gong cleanses the body of toxins, restores energy, and reduces stress and anxiety. It helps maintain a healthy and active lifestyle. It also improves athletic performance by sharpening focus, balance and relaxation.

Qi Gong is accessible to people of all ages. In fact, it is particularly beneficial to the elderly and those with impaired motor skills. Moreover, no special clothes or equipment are required, and you can practice at home.

Balance is the principle of health. As the internal organs come into balance, health improves, and the Mind becomes tranquil. Practicing Qi Gong harmonizes the Qi in the organs, improves blood circulation, enhances our immune system and delays aging.

The most important signs are sounder sleep, better recovery from stress or disease, a clearer Mind, more energy and flexibility, and a general calmness and youthful appearance. The practice of Qi Gong brings many benefits:

- Promotes relaxation
- Reduces stress
- Improves concentration
- Cultivates mental alertness
- Helps improve balance
- Strengthens the immune system
- Lowers the demand for oxygen
- Increases the Lungs capacity to absorb oxygen
- Helps normalize the white blood count
- Promotes circulation of Qi and blood
- Lowers blood pressure, pulse and metabolic rates
- Raises endocrine systems capabilities
- Repairs and adjusts the nervous system
- Develops intelligence potential
- Strengthens muscles and bones
- Produces an optimistic and happy attitude towards life

How to Cultivate Qi

"Ideal health is a state of no energy blockages, where energy flows freely throughout the body. There is no physical, energetic or emotional conflict in the body. Perfect balance exists." Adam (Energy Healer)

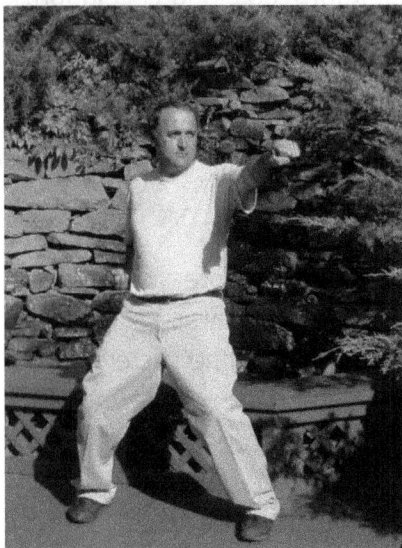

During a Qi Gong training session one of my instructors explained that Qi could be very volatile. "Treat it gently much like you would hold a newborn baby. Otherwise it could disappear as quickly as it appeared," he indicated.

We are essentially energy beings. If Qi flows abundantly and freely in our bodies, we will enjoy a healthy and vibrant life. If Qi stagnates or is depleted, illness and eventually death will follow.

The free flow of Qi can be blocked because of an injury. Strong emotions and a stressful lifestyle can also hinder the flow of Qi. Hereditary factors play an important role in determining how much essential Qi a person has at birth.

As we grow older the body weakens, moving from a Yang to a Yin state of energy. During the autumn of our lives, as our physical body weakens, the ability to cultivate Qi becomes even more important in maintaining health and longevity.

We can cultivate Qi using several methods. Qi Gong teaches relaxation, posture, gentle movement, breath, healing sounds, and self-massage to strengthen the body and the Mind. Advanced practitioners can readily feel the Qi between the palms of the hands, move it to different parts of the body, and exchange Qi with nature and distant galaxies.

With over 3,000 years of history, Qi Gong has grown to include thousands of different styles. A lifetime would be insufficient to master the many variances of this healing art. Nevertheless, there are common underpinnings in all Qi Gong styles that are essential to the practice of the art and distinguish Qi Gong from many other exercise forms being practiced today.

On a technical level the combination of movement and stillness, breath and Mind-Moving-Qi are very distinct. But it is the spirit of heart-felt awareness that truly distinguishes Qi Gong from many other disciplines. True Qi Gong has no form. It expresses itself from the Heart.

As Grand Master Shih has said many times to his students, "do good things for others and be helpful. Your kindness will bring good things to you. Your body and Heart will attain health and longevity. Empty your Mind and embrace nothingness. This is the abundant energy of your life source."

I will attempt to provide you with the basic tools to embark on the path of Qi Gong. Everything starts and ends with the basics. The more you practice the more you will understand, the more you will grow your Qi.

Everyone can benefit from Qi Gong. But like all disciplines it demands commitment, regular practice, and often commands a change of lifestyle. Start now with this advice from Grand Master Shih: **Relax, Be Happy, and Smile from the Heart.**

Energy Anatomy

To be successful in the treatment of disorders and disease, medical professionals need a strong foundation in disciplines such as anatomy, neurology, physiology and pathology. To better understand how to cultivate Qi, it is equally important to understand the anatomy of the energy body. This discipline touches upon many areas such as Yin and Yang, the Three Dantians, Three Treasures, the body's Bio-Energy Field or Aura, Twelve Chakras, Twelve Regular Meridians, and Eight Extraordinary Meridians.

Yin and Yang

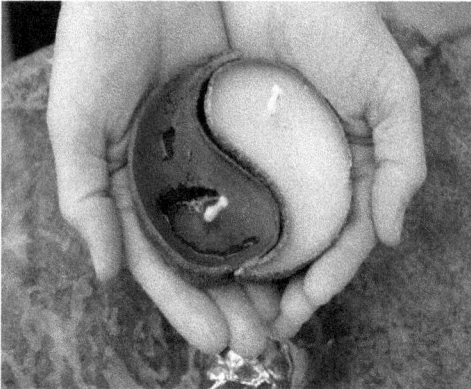

Qi or life energy is made up of two complimentary and opposing forces called Yin and Yang. Yin and Yang are two sides of the same Qi coin. One cannot exist without the other.

Yin is dark, passive and feminine. Yang is light, active, and masculine. All things are made of both Yin and Yang that naturally balance each other. Yin continually changes into Yang, and Yang into Yin. Their interaction creates life.

The Chinese characters for Yin and Yang are related to the image of a hill. One side of the hill is in the shade while the other is in the sunlight. The character Yin indicates the shady side of the hill while the character Yang indicates the sunny side of the hill.

The Moon is Yin. The Sun is Yang. Yin conserves, contracts and descends. Yang transforms, expands and rises. Yin is inside and restful. Yang is outside and active. Yin is opposite to Yang. They are two stages of a cyclical movement one constantly changing into the other, such as day turning into night, summer into winter, and growth into decay. Everything contains the seeds of its opposite.

The Daoist classic "Dao De Jing" by Lao Zi illustrates this point: "In order to contract, it is necessary to first expand." Yin and Yang are in a constant state of dynamic balance.

Understanding the principles of Yin and Yang has an application in the practice of Qi Gong. For example, excessive work (Yang) without rest leads to extreme deficiency (Yin) of the body's energies. Excessive worrying (Yang) depletes the (Yin) energy of the body. Excessive sexual activity (Yang) depletes the Essence (Yin).

A standing posture helps descend Yang Qi. It lowers High Blood Pressure and helps resolve digestive issues related to rebellious Qi. Palms facing up raise Yang Qi and help normalize Low Blood Pressure. External movements develop Yang Qi while internal movements develop Yin Qi.

Yin and Yang are in a constant state of waxing and waning. If this waxing and waning exceeds the body's normal energetic limits and loses its dynamic equilibrium, Deficient or Excess Yin or Yang will occur, leading to the development of abnormalities and illness.

Three Dantians

According to Medical Qi Gong, humans have three important energy centers called the Upper, Middle and Lower Dantians. A Dantian or Elixir Field is where Qi is gathered, stored and transformed.

The Three Dantians communicate with each other via the Taiji Pole. This energetic channel flows from the Bai Hui point on the crown of the head, through the center core of the body, to the center of the perineum at the Hui Yin. The Three Dantians connect smaller energy gates called Chakras, or spiraling wheels of energy, that originate from the Taiji Pole and spiral outwards into the body's energy field.

The Lower Dantian or House of the Earthly Realm is the center of physical strength and stamina. It is here that Yuan Qi originates and resides. This Dantian is in the lower abdomen in the center of the triangle formed by joining the point located at the navel called Shen Que or Spirit Gate, the point on the lower back called Mingmen or

Gate of Fire, and the center of the perineum called Hui Yin or Meeting of Yin.

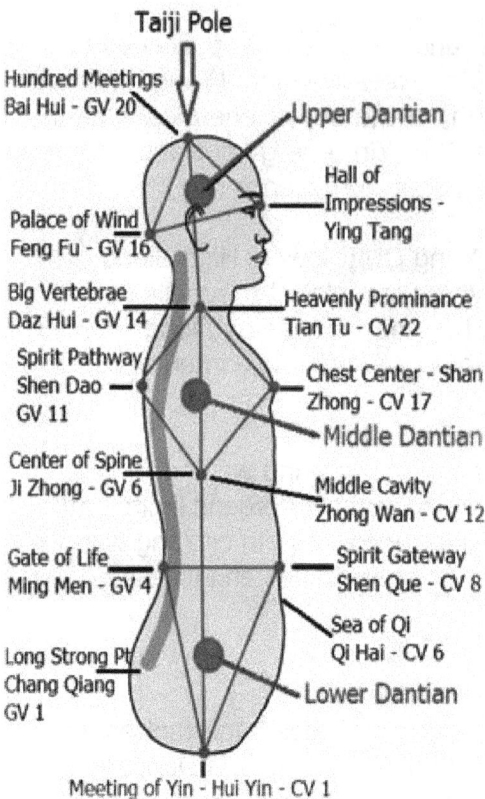

Taiji Pole

Hundred Meetings
Bai Hui - GV 20

Upper Dantian

Hall of
Impressions -
Ying Tang

Palace of Wind
Feng Fu - GV 16

Big Vertebrae
Daz Hui - GV 14

Heavenly Prominance
Tian Tu - CV 22

Spirit Pathway
Shen Dao -
GV 11

Chest Center - Shan
Zhong - CV 17

Middle Dantian

Center of Spine
Ji Zhong - GV 6

Middle Cavity
Zhong Wan - CV 12

Gate of Life
Ming Men - GV 4

Spirit Gateway
Shen Que - CV 8

Sea of Qi
Qi Hai - CV 6

Long Strong Pt
Chang Qiang
GV 1

Lower Dantian

Meeting of Yin - Hui Yin - CV 1

The triangle faces downward allowing the Lower Dantian to gather denser Yin energy from the Earth. Earth energy is required to help ground the Qi Gong practitioner, balancing the active Yang energy gathered during the practice of Qi Gong. Collecting energy in the Lower Dantian increases awareness and intuitive perception leading to naturally occurring body movements.

This zone is primarily responsible for physical strength, sexual vitality and overall health. Qi Gong practice encourages returning to the source or Lower Dantian to help strengthen the root of the body's energy.

The Middle Dantian or House of the Human Realm gathers lighter less substantial Yin and Yang energy from Heaven and Earth, creating a distinct kind of emotional energy normally associated with human beings.

This reservoir for mental and emotional energy reflects the Heart's energetic capacity to express feelings and show compassion. It is associated with storing Shen or Spirit, with respiration, and with the health of the internal organs, in particular the thymus gland. Its energy is more akin to vibration.

The Middle Dantian's field of energy naturally extends into both palms. It is the main region responsible for the refinement of vitality or Qi into Spirit. It is located at the level of the Heart in the mid chest area. It forms a square with its four extremities defined by six acupuncture points.

Its lower front point is located on the abdomen half way between the navel and sternocostal angle called the Zhong Wan or Middle Cavity. The front center point of the Middle Dantian is located at the center of the chest, on the midline of the sternum called the Shan Zhong or Chest Center. The upper front point of the Middle Dantian is located at the suprasternal notch called the Tian Tu or Heavenly Prominence.

The upper back point is located above the 1st thoracic vertebrae called the Daz Hui or Great Vertebrae. The mid back point is located above the 6th thoracic vertebrae between the scapula called Shen Dao or Spirit Pathway. The lower point is located above the 12th thoracic vertebrae called Ji Zhong or Center of Spine.

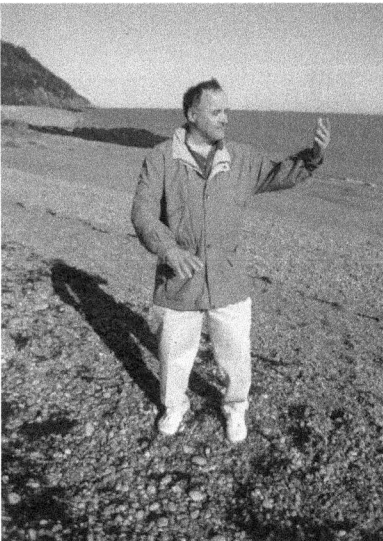

The Upper Dantian or House of the Spirit Realm collects energy from the Universe - Sun, Moon, Planets and Stars, and represents your spiritual aspect. This energy is more akin to vapor. It is associated with light and is Yang in nature. It is the least substantial of all three energies. This is where the wisdom Mind perceives subtler vibrations and frequencies emitted by the earth, planets and stars. Psychic perceptions and intuitive knowing that transcend time and space emanate from this region.

The center of the Upper Dantian is in the pineal gland, a small endocrine gland, located near to the center of the brain between the two hemispheres. The pineal gland produces melatonin, a hormone that affects the modulation of wake/sleep patterns and photoperiodic (seasonal) functions. Mystical traditions and esoteric schools have long known this area in the middle of the brain to be the connecting link between the physical and spiritual worlds.

The Upper Dantian is shaped like a pyramid facing upward. This allows it to gather energy from the Stars. It transforms Shen into Wuji or the openness of infinite space.

The front gate of the Upper Dantian is located at the center of the eyebrows called the Yin Tang or Hall of Impressions, the back gate in a depression immediately below the external occipital protuberance called the Feng Fu or Palace of Wind, and the highest gate is located at the top or crown of the head called the Bai Hui or Hundred Meetings.

The combined energetic qualities of all three Dantians form the foundation for all psychic perceptions. Pure intent and a quiet Mind are required to favor accurate psychic perceptions and true communication with the higher self. Each Dantian collects energy from the Universe and redistributes it to all the internal organs. In turn, this energy is projected into the body's Wei Qi field. **Wei Qi** *(pronounced "whey chee")* translates as **"protective energy."**

In Traditional Chinese Medicine, the Wei Qi field is limited to the surface of the body, circulating between the skin and the muscles. In Medical Qi Gong, the Wei Qi field includes the three external layers of the body's subtle energy fields sometimes referred to as the body's Bio-Energy Field or Aura.

The Wei Qi field surrounds, flows through and extends from the human body. The energy from the Lower Dantian projects about an inch away from the body in the physical field, the Middle Dantian projects to about a foot and a half away from the body in the emotional field, and the Upper Dantian projects several feet away from the body in the intuitive or spiritual field.

Three Treasures: Jing, Qi, Shen

The body is primarily composed of subtle energy. This subtle energy manifests eventually as the physical body. A traditional way of describing this condition is with the three treasures, Jing, Qi and Shen. The three treasures are the fundamental energies required for human life. They form the essential trinity of our physical manifestation.

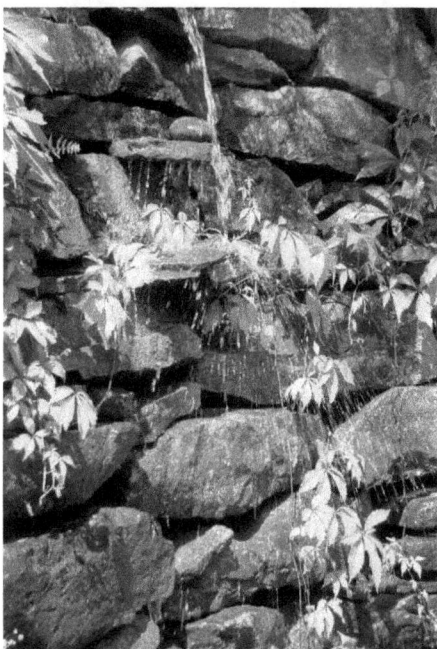

The Three Dantians store, cultivate and transform Shen, Qi and Jing energy. The Lower Dantian transforms Jing into Qi. The Middle Dantian transforms Qi into Shen or spiritual consciousness, and the Upper Dantian transforms Shen into Wuji, emptiness, or void energy.

Shen is generally translated as the Spirit-Mind that maintains form and consciousness. When it is disordered, the form of a person changes and consciousness becomes disturbed. It is commonly believed in the healing and martial arts that the Shen or Mind leads the Qi.

Qi is the active force that animates the physical body and its vital functions. It is a person's vitality that causes others to describe them as energetic and alive. A person may have a strong Shen or Mind, but their body may not be very alive. When the body has Qi the person is obviously energetic.

Qi can be acquired from the food we eat and the air we breathe. Of course, the practice of Qi Gong helps cultivate Qi, strengthening both the body and the Mind. The abundance of acquired Qi is influenced by how we live. Physical exercise, proper diet, and healthy emotions can help build more Qi. Excessive sex, unbalanced emotions, over work and over thinking depletes Qi. Qi refines the Jing.

Jing is the underlying physical essence, a mixture of constitutional or genetic force that is associated with the sexual function and vitality of a person but without the clearly obvious active energetic presence of Qi. It is often associated with the perception of depth or a quality of endurance of a person.

In Traditional Chinese Medicine, it is believed that Jing Qi is largely determined at birth by a person's genetic makeup, as well as by the overall health and age of our parents at the time of conception. If Jing Qi is weak at birth or depleted afterwards because of bad nutrition, overwork or stress, it is very difficult to rebuild.

These three qualities, Jing-Qi-Shen, form the basis of an individual. They interact to mutually support each other. The practice of Qi Gong helps build strong Jing-Qi-Shen.

First solidify the root energy or essential essence located in the lower Dantian. By putting the Mind in the lower Dantian energy will come. Just place the Mind there naturally, relaxed and without thoughts. It is believed that by keeping the Shen in the body, with no desires and thoughts, one can live up to 125 years.

The 12 Chakras

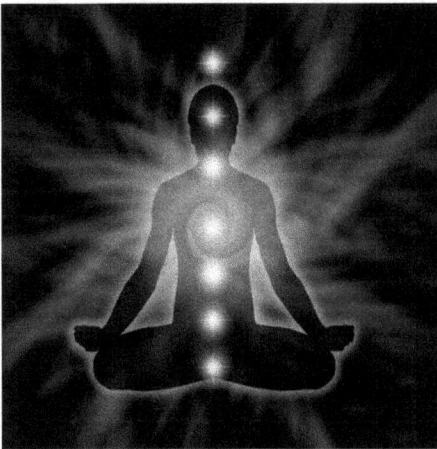

Ancient mystics claimed they could see wheels of light or energy spinning outward from various points on the body. These wheels of light are now called Chakras, which is a Sanskrit word that means wheel or disk. Each Chakra extends its energy vortex outward from the body's Tai Chi pole into the Wei Qi field or Aura.

In her book, Healing Touch, a Guidebook for Practitioners, Dorothea Hover-Kramer, compares Chakras to energy transfer stations that allow the inflow of Qi from the Universe and outflow of excessive energy from the body.

According to Dr. Jerry Alan Johnson, author of Chinese Medical Qi Gong Therapy - A Comprehensive Clinical Text, Chakras also reflect the various aspects of consciousness from the past, present and future.

The chakras are vertically aligned running from the base of the spine to the crown of the head. The five front Chakra gates are located on the front centerline of the body. They are responsible for emotions as they are related to the Shen or Spirit, and the Heart Fire. The five back Chakras are located along the spinal column. They are responsible for willpower and determination.

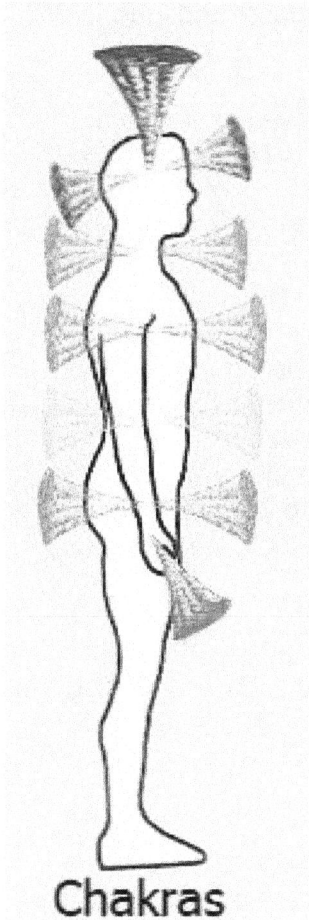

Chakras

The Root Chakra located at the Hui Yin in the center of the perineum absorbs Qi from the earth energizing the Taiji Pole or central energetic core of the body. The root Chakra is associated with the instinct of survival. Its malfunction can cause fear, which can lead to lower back pain, sciatica, constipation, hemorrhoids, rectal tumors, knee problems, immune related disorders, and varicose veins.

The Sacral Chakra front gate is located just below the navel with the back gate along the lumbar spine below the second lumbar vertebrae. This Chakra is the center for sexuality, sensuality, hunger for power and financial issues. It supplies the sexual organs and the immune system with energy. Malfunction of this Chakra can cause chronic lower back pain, frigidity or impotence as well as Kidney, uterine and urinary problems.

The Solar Plexus Chakra Front Gate is located half way between the navel and the tip of the sternum with the back gate at the middle of the spine below the eleventh thoracic vertebrae. It is a gathering point for gut-felt intuition, personal power and self-image.

Severe anger and emotional pain related to fear of rejection are often stored here. Energetic malfunctions can cause ulcers, hypoglycemia, chronic or acute indigestion, and diabetes as well as Liver and adrenal problems.

The Heart Chakra Front Gate is located at the center of the chest with the back gate between the scapula below the fifth thoracic vertebrae. This Chakra is a gathering point for love, compassion, empathy, clairsentience and intuition. Energy malfunctions can cause congestive heart failure, heart attacks, breast cancer and lung disease.

The Throat Chakra front gate is located just above the hollow of the throat with the back gate at the base of the neck below the seventh cervical vertebrae. This gate's energy is related to personal and divine will, and communication. When it opens there is an urge to sing and chant.

Energetic malfunctions can cause a knot within the throat, sore throat, stiff neck, thyroid problems, TMJ, and swollen glands. The opening of this gate can release unexpressed grief or anger.

The Brow Chakra Front gate is located between the eyebrows with the back gate in a depression directly superior to the external occipital protuberance. This is the center of intuition, clairvoyance and energy projection.

The Brow Chakra is responsible for mental telepathy and the ability to see auras. Energetic malfunctions can result in headaches, eye strain, pain around the eyes, distorted or blurred vision, blindness, deafness, inaccurate interpretations of events, projection of personal fears onto others and recurring nightmares.

The Crown Chakra located at the crown of the head absorbs Universal Qi and light into the body, energizing the center core. This energy center is associated with higher knowledge, understanding, pure intuition and ecstasy. Its malfunction results in confusion, apathy, alienation, boredom, depression and incomprehension.

Minor Chakras are located at all the joints of the body such as the hips, knees, ankles, feet, shoulders, elbows, wrists and hands, as well as at hundreds of points located along the energy channels or meridians that circulate throughout the whole body. As seen in the following chart, each major Chakra is associated with an element, sound, color and functional quality.

Chakra	Element	Sound	Color	Associated with
Root	Earth	Bumblebee	Red	Survival Instincts
Sacral	Water	Melody of a Wooden Flute	Orange	Sexuality
Solar Plexus	Fire	Stringed Instruments	Yellow	Self-image & Staying Power
Heart	Wind	Bells	Emerald Green	Compassion
Throat	Sound	Wind Blowing	Bright Blue	Communication Clairaudience
Brow	Light	Waves Crashing on the Beach	Indigo Blue	Clairvoyant Seeing Mental Imagery
Crown	Infinite Space	"Aum" or "Om"	Purple, lavender, white to silver	Oneness & Higher Knowledge

The Aura or Bio-Energy Field

Every living thing, from plants, to animals, trees, leaves and cells are surrounded by a bio-energy field or aura. The word "aura" literally means "breeze". Scientific research has found that auras are an electromagnetic field that resonates at different frequencies of light. The Japanese physicist Motoyama has measured the human bioelectric field at various distances from the body with delicate scientific instruments.

The aura circulates four to five feet around the physical body and traverses the body. It manifests itself as shimmering layers of luminous, colored energy. People with special abilities can see the energy field around objects and living beings through their peripheral field of vision.

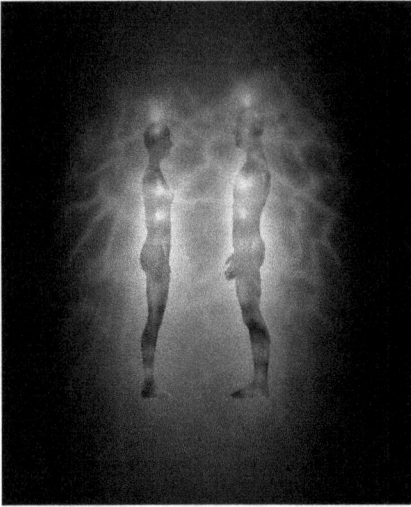

The colors, which are part of the body's radiant energy, are constantly in motion, reacting to thoughts, emotions, and environmental influences. The emotions and thoughts that vibrate within the field serve to transmit feelings and information to other human beings.

The strength of the aura is directly connected to the level of health and vitality of the person. A person who is physically and mentally healthy with positive spiritual energies has a bigger and brighter aura in contrast to that of an unhealthy person.

Many texts, both ancient and modern, describe the various layers of the bio-energy field. For this discussion, we will study three layers of significance for Qi Gong.

1. Physical Layer: This layer is closely associated with the physical body. It interfaces with the Lower Dantian and extends 2 to 12 inches from the skin. It is often associated with energy-balancing work.

2. Emotional Layer: This level, which extends outward about a foot and a half from the body, holds the individual's affective, feeling energy, and interfaces with the Middle Dantian.

3. Intuitive or Spiritual Layer: This level, which extends several feet away from the body, relates to the spiritual and intuitive dimensions of the individual and interfaces with the Upper Dantian.

Imbalance or dysfunction may occur in any of the layers of the energy field.

Dysfunction in the physical layer can lead overtime to physical symptoms and disease. Dysfunction in the emotional layer constricts the energy leading to such conditions as depression or despair. Dysfunction in the spiritual or intuitive layer is the most devastating as it impacts all other layers. It is experienced as a loss of purpose or sense of hope.

The Twelve Regular Meridians

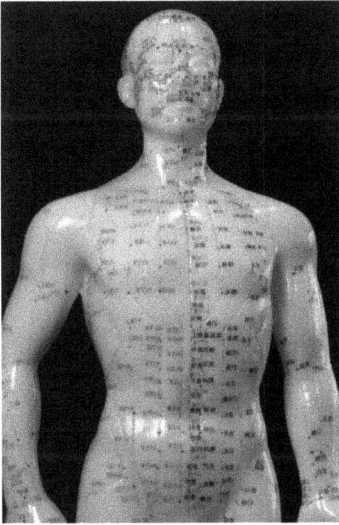

Meridians are channels of energy that run in regular patterns through the body and over its surface. They are like cosmic doors that open and close allowing the body to communicate with the energies of the Universe.

Like rivers they irrigate and nourish the tissues and organs. Any obstruction in their movement can cause stagnant energy to build up adversely affecting overall health. The flow of energy in the meridians can be reestablished by stretching fascial tissue, needling, applying pressure, or extending energy to the appropriate acupuncture points situated along the meridians.

Western science believes that needling the acupuncture points stimulates the nervous system releasing chemicals and hormones which influence the body's own internal regulating system. The improved energy and biochemical balance produced by acupuncture stimulates the body's natural healing abilities and promotes physical and emotional well-being.

There are 12 Regular Meridians, and each is associated with an organ or functional unit. The twelve meridians are named according to their corresponding organs, limb positions and Yin and Yang properties.

Yin meridians provide strength and stability while Yang meridians consolidate defenses on the exterior of the body.

The 12 Regular Meridians include:

- Three arm Yin meridians (Lung, Pericardium, Heart)
- Three arm Yang meridians (Large Intestine, Triple Burner, Small Intestine)
- Three leg Yin meridians (Spleen, Liver, Kidney)
- Three leg Yang meridians (Stomach, Gall Bladder, Bladder)

The Triple Burner and the Pericardium, located on the arms, do not refer to anatomical structures. Traditional Chinese Medicine (TCM) considers them as functional units.

The Eight Extraordinary Meridians

The Eight Extraordinary Meridians are the body's deepest level of energetic structuring. These meridians are the first to form in utero and are carriers of Yuan Qi - the ancestral energy which corresponds to our genetic inheritance.

They function as deep reservoirs from which the twelve main meridians are replenished, and into which the latter can drain their excesses. Other names for these Eight Extraordinary Meridians include: The Eight Curious Vessels, the Eight Marvelous Meridians, and the Eight Irregular Vessels.

The specific meridians belonging to the "Eight Extras" family are:
- Du Mai (Governing Vessel)
- Ren Mai (Conception Vessel)
- Chong Mai (Penetrating Vessel)
- Dai Mai (Belt Channel or Girdling Vessel)
- Yang Qiao Mai (Yang Motility or Heel Vessel)
- Yin Qiao Mai (Yin Motility or Heel Vessel)
- Yang Wei Mai (Yang Regulating or Linking Vessel)
- Yin Wei Mai (Yin Regulating or Linking Vessel)

In TCM, the Eight Extraordinary Vessels are typically used in pairs: Ren with Yin Qiao, Du with Yang Qiao, Chong with Yin Wei, and Dai with Yang Wei. Of these eight meridians, only the Ren and the Du

34

have their own acupuncture points. The other six utilize points to activate the Qi that belong to the twelve Regular Meridians.

The most important of the Eight Extraordinary Meridians for Qi Gong practice are the Du Mai (Governing Vessel), the Ren Mai (Conception Vessel), the Chong Mai (Penetrating Vessel), and the Dai Mai (Belt Channel).

The Du Mai flows from the tip of the coccyx up the spine, over the head, and ends in the upper part of the mouth. The Ren Mai flows from the perineum up along the front mid-line of the torso and ends in the lower mouth.

In the Microcosmic Orbit practice, the Ren and the Du meridians are linked into a single continuous circuit. The Qi moves from the Lower Dantian up the spine along the Du Mai, then down the Ren Mai on the front of the body to the perineum. This is how energy circulated when we were in our mother's womb.

The Chong Meridian flows vertically deep within the body, along the front of the spine, and is most closely associated with Yuan Qi. The Chong Mai has a close resonance with – if not an actual equivalence to - the Shushumna Nadi described in Hindu Yogic traditions. It is our energetic core or Tai Chi Pole.

The Dai Mai circles the waist and is the only horizontally-flowing meridian. As such, it acts as a kind of "belt" - containing the other vertically-flowing meridians. It circulates energy between the upper and lower parts of the body while keeping our shape and holding our form.

Key Points in Qi Gong Practice

Above all:

- **Remain rooted to the earth**
- **Suspend the Crown of the head from above**
- **Open the body to the Universe**
- **Smile from the Heart**
- **Embrace all things**

Mastery of the basics through sustained practice is required in all art forms. Embracing the concept of cultivation, "a gradual growth due to consistent, intentional activity", is extremely important to the successful practice of Qi Gong.

Important points in Qi Gong practice involve Body Posture, Body Movement, Breath and Mind Moving Qi.

Body Posture

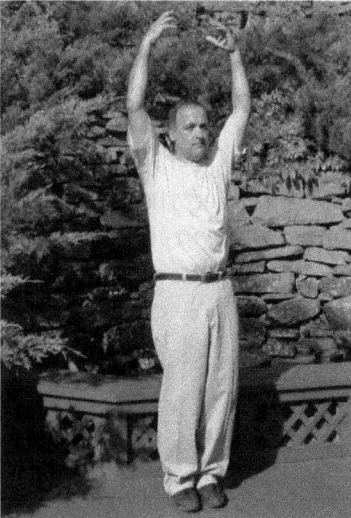

All Qi Gong forms begin with correct posture. When the body is properly aligned energy can flow more abundantly. The objective of good posture is to allow the bones of the skeleton to stack up one upon the other in perfect balance thus allowing the body to stay upright with little or no effort. The energy thus liberated can be used to promote a healthy body and a healthy Mind.

Good posture starts at the feet, the body's foundation. Relax and let the weight of the body flow downwards towards the centre of the earth, while maintaining extension upwards through the Crown Point located on the top of the head.

The use of specific postures for changing consciousness and correcting Qi flow through the body is very ancient. The physical position of the body plays a very important role in the functioning of all aspects of the physiological process.

The most important aspect of posture is the position of the spine. The spine has been called the ridgepole of the Universe. The ridgepole is the central post around which the rest of the body structure is built.

The spine functions as the main vertical support for all the internal organs. It is also the major pathway for the nervous system. It provides the energetic link for the flow of Qi into the internal organs from the rear of the body. The spine not only innervates the organs but also relays sensory and motor information to the brain.

An erect spine and stable lower body structure help the body resist the constant pull of gravity. This benefits the overall energy of the body by reducing the activity level of the muscles involved in maintaining an upright posture.

Correct posture allows for a free flow of the Qi and Blood. It helps prevent many musculoskeletal degenerative diseases that are caused by chronic overuse and misaligned joints. This adds years to a person's quality of life.

A good stance and posture reflect a proper state of Mind. If body posture is incorrect, then the Mind is not peaceful. Knowledge about posture can help a person correct various health problems. One can adopt different postures to develop different states of Mind and different types of Qi, thus influencing the health of the body and the Mind.

There are three main body positions used in practice: sitting, standing and lying down. Qi Gong can also be practiced while walking or running. Each body posture must respect basic principles of keeping the head erect, the body aligned and rooted to the earth, the joints open and relaxed.

Standing

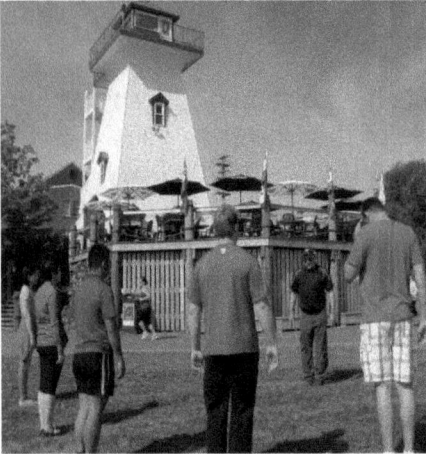

- Stand in an upright position, feet together, hip width apart or shoulder width apart
- Look far into the distance. Keep eyes soft and open, or half-closed
- Let the chin move inwards towards the Adams Apple, gently lifting the Adams Apple, with the Crown of the head suspended from above
- Open the space between the shoulder blades
- Gently place the tip of the tongue on the upper palate behind the front teeth
- Arms hang down and slightly away from the sides of the body, or on occasion hold an energy ball in front of the navel or mid chest area
- Gently move the abdomen inward towards the lower back or Ming Men
- Gently lift the anus
- Tilt the hips forward to straighten the lower back
- Knees are straight but soft
- Feet are rooted deep into the earth, with the body weight 70% on the heels
- Place the Mind in the center of the abdomen

In the standing posture, the feet are parallel to each other usually shoulder width apart to balance Yin and Yang energies from side to side and back to front. The arms hang usually to the side, palms open and facing the lateral aspect of the body. If your energy is too Yang you need to stand. The standing posture benefits people over 40 as it helps reduce High Blood Pressure and calms the digestive system.

Keeping the knees bent slightly and tailbone curled under as if sitting on a chair guides the energy down towards the earth. Standing with the arms to the side and the Mind placed in the center of abdomen helps reduce high blood pressure, heart palpitations, headaches and heart disease.

Palms facing down reduce High Blood Pressure or excessive Yang. Palms facing up reduce Low Blood Pressure or excessive Yin. Palms facing the abdomen with a deep stance develop strong abdominal Qi.

Sitting

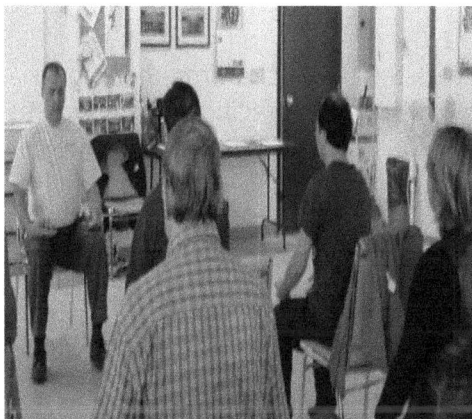

When practicing Qi Gong, you can sit in a chair, or on the floor. There are two major postures when sitting on the floor: Lotus or Half Lotus which is a cross-legged posture common in Yoga, and Seiza or kneeling with the lower legs folded underneath the thighs, while resting the buttocks on the heels, common in the Japanese martial arts.

When sitting on a chair, the hips are located on the front third of the chair so that the reproductive organs are not constricted. This enables the energy to move more freely in the Microcosmic Orbit which is comprised of the Governing and Conception Meridians.

People with weak backs can use the back of the chair for support. The feet are shoulder width apart, parallel to each other, with the lower legs perpendicular to the earth.

When in a Lotus or Half Lotus position the hips are slightly elevated by sitting on a firm cushion with the weight of the body on the sit bones (Ischial Tuberosity). The Lotus or Half Lotus position helps gain quietness and is more powerful in activating the Lower Dantian located in the center of the abdomen.

Sitting in Seiza develops a strong center or Hara. It is a very relaxing posture that helps strengthen the knees and open the Stomach meridian located in the lower legs. When sitting in Seiza, we often place a Yoga block on its side between the feet under the buttocks to help reduce pressure on the knees.

Most people sit when they practice. If your energy is too Yin or in a weakened state, sit or lie down. The sitting position, with palms on the thighs facing down or up, facilitates breathing and prevents asthma and coughing.

If suffering from High Blood pressure stand with the arms hanging down the sides of the body or sit with the palms facing downwards to help lower the Qi.

Lying Down

When lying on the back, use a support to elevate the head four inches up from the floor so you can see the navel. This is good for the Stomach and Spleen. If the Stomach drops down, raise the hip a little to correct the problem. Lying on the right side is more appropriate than lying on the left side. Left lying is not good for the Heart as it restricts the flow of energy.

When side lying, the lower leg is straight, the upper leg is bent slightly over the lower leg. The lower hand is placed in front of the forehead. This position is good for the Heart, Stomach and Spleen. Both sitting and half-lying positions are good for asthma.

Body Movement

Together with proper posture, repetitive movement releases stagnant Qi and blood from blocked areas of the body. By mechanically squeezing and stretching connective tissue and muscles and by opening joints, repetitive movement stimulates the flow of Qi and Blood.

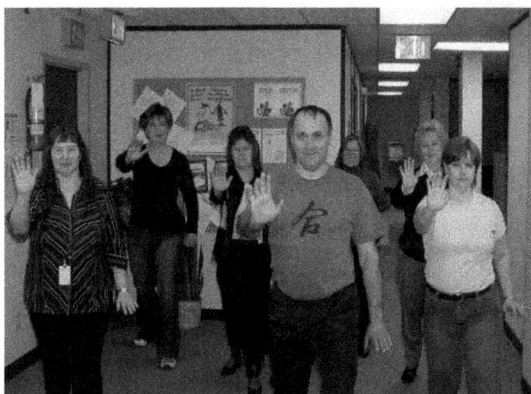

Qi tends to stagnate in areas of the body that harbor muscle tension. Gentle repetitive movement with conscious awareness facilitates the release of this tension and the rebalancing of the flow of Qi through the meridians or energy channels.

Repetitive, slow movement facilitates the function of the autonomic nervous system by lowering sympathetic nervous system activity and raising parasympathetic nervous system activity. These two parts of the autonomic nervous system function to regulate and control a wide variety of physiological activities that are vital to the healthy functioning of the respiratory, digestive, urogenital and reproductive systems.

The lymphatic system is a very low-pressure system. The rhythmic contraction/relaxation of the muscles increases the flow of lymph and intracellular fluids. It also compresses the capillary system that brings nutrients and oxygen to the cells and takes away carbon dioxide and waste products of cellular metabolism. This literally squeezes and forces the blood through the low-pressure end of the circulatory system, more efficiently feeding and nourishing the cells of the body.

Body movement also plays an important role in strengthening the immune system by removing dead bacteria and the cellular debris, and by mobilizing lymphocytes to help fight infection.

Breath

Breathing is the first thing you do when you leave the security of your mother's womb and the last thing you do before you die. Paying attention to breath pays big dividends, as breath and Qi are one. The pattern of the breath also reflects the spirit of the style of Qi Gong being practiced.

Ingrained patterns of behaviour caused by fear or insecurity often limit the body's ability to breathe naturally. With proper training adults can regain the natural breath they had when they were born and thus benefit from a greater sense of tranquility and vitality.

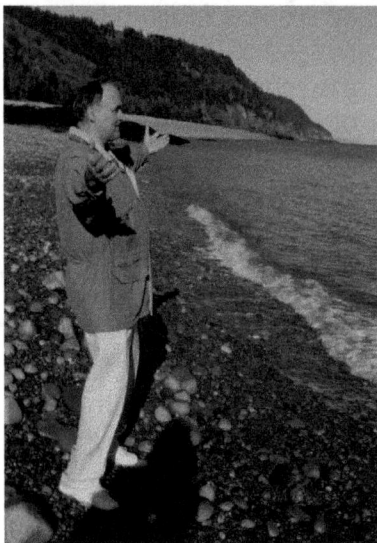

Many areas inside the body do not move, often limiting the circulation of Blood and Qi. Natural breathing moves the diaphragms that massage internal organs, improving Blood and Qi circulation. The increased energy flow helps the whole body stay healthy.

In Traditional Chinese Medicine, the Lungs govern Qi and respiration. They disperse or move the Qi through the body via the energy channels and their collaterals. The Lungs cause the Qi to descend to the lower part of the body, activating and fueling the vital physiological functions associated with digestion and the formation of Blood. The Kidneys assist the Lungs in holding and stabilizing the breath on inhalation.

The Lungs also rule the surface of the body and the Wei Qi, or protective Qi that, according to Traditional Chinese Medicine, moves just below the surface of the skin, and according to Medical Qi Gong extends into the three external layers of the body's Aura. It forms a protective barrier to the invasion of the body by external pathogenic agents.

The concept of cultivation is especially important in breathing exercises since they are the quickest acting and can produce the strongest initial response of any of the principles of Qi Gong.

Proper breathing helps relax the body. It brings much needed oxygen into the cells and helps cleanse the body of toxins. It massages the internal organs and encourages proper posture. Breath harmonises body and Spirit into one action, one being.

Various systems of breathing affect the body differently. Some favor relaxation, others stimulate Qi, while others release toxins. The most common types of breathing are Relaxed Belly Breathing or "Post-Natal Breathing", Reverse Belly Breathing or "Pre-Natal Breathing", Varying Length Breathing or alternating cycles of longer-shorter breathing, and Pulsating Breath.

Post-Natal or Relaxed Belly Breathing

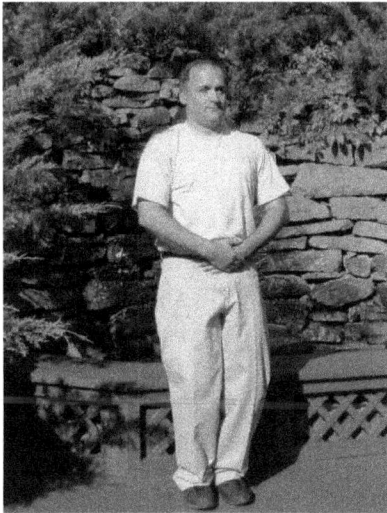

Post-Natal or Relaxed Belly Breathing promotes relaxation and helps detoxify the body. When air is drawn into the Lungs, the area around the abdomen and lower back expands, and the chest lifts and expands. As the air leaves the Lungs, the chest and shoulders fall, and the abdomen naturally contracts.

Two of the major diaphragms active in breathing are the perineum located between the anus and sexual organs and the thoracic diaphragm located below the Lungs separating the chest from the abdomen. On inhalation both diaphragms drop downward, drawing air into the Lung cavities. On exhalation, the diaphragms release, moving upwards pushing air out of the Lungs.

The objective of Relaxed Belly Breathing is to become more relaxed and alert. Inhale about 70 percent of Lung capacity to avoid stressing the upper part of the body, and exhale 100 percent to expel stagnant Qi and toxins from the body.

Natural breathing is like a wave, undulating up and down the body, in a wonderfully invigorating movement. The breath moves in and out like an unbroken thread. On the top of the inhalation it slows and

43

changes direction much like waves moving up a sandy beach only to return to the ocean. On the bottom of the exhalation, as the cycle continues, it also slows and changes direction.

To help deepen the breath, stretch out the down beat as much as possible while staying calm and relaxed. The inhalation will rise on its own from the quietness that occupies the space between exhalation and inhalation.

A normal person breathes from 16 to 18 times a minute. Qi Gong practitioners can breathe four times per minute without effort. With more extensive training the breathing rhythm can be reduced to two breaths per minute, creating an intense feeling of relaxation.

This increases awareness of energy, the depth of practice and one's ability to direct the flow of Qi improving health and vitality. Observing breath helps calm the Mind and encourages the flow of energy or Qi.

Relaxed Belly breathing lowers blood pressure, activates peristalsis and increases venous return of oxygenated blood. This improves the overall level of oxygen in the blood. It also draws the Qi down into the lower part of the body, which helps to relax the Mind and build Qi in the lower Dantian.

Focused lower belly breathing also strengthens the Kidneys and the Mingmen Fire. The Kidneys in Traditional Chinese Medicine are the activating Yang element for the Spleen and the Lungs, thereby supporting the digestive and respiratory functions.

Breathing that is focused in the upper chest increases blood pressure and stimulates the Heart and Lungs to move the Blood and Qi more quickly and with greater force through the body. This can be very helpful for persons with low blood pressure and mental dullness due to sluggish circulation of Blood and Qi.

Start practicing with Relaxed Belly Breathing. This is good for the Spleen and Stomach. This is important as acquired Qi comes in part from these two organs. This type of breathing also exercises the internal organs helping the whole body. As it has positive effects on circulation, it helps correct blood pressure problems and nervousness. When this energy moves, many health problems disappear.

Pre-Natal or Reverse Belly Breathing

During Post-Natal Breathing or Relaxed Belly Breathing, when inhaling, the lower abdomen expands, and the abdominal muscles are relaxed. When exhaling the lower abdomen contracts, moving toward the center of the body as the diaphragms and the intra-abdominal pressure are released.

Pre-Natal Breathing or Reverse Belly Breathing uses an active contraction of the abdominal muscles upon inhalation to compress the abdominal cavity. These muscles then relax upon exhalation and the lower abdomen protrudes. Sometimes the muscles of the lower cavity around the anus and genitals are actively contracted on inhalation to provide added pressure in the abdominal cavity.

Reverse Belly Breathing can powerfully move the Qi through the energy channels in an upward direction. It massages the internal organs creating heat and energy, strengthening Jing Qi, and helping resolve lower body issues such as a prolapsed anus, uterus or vagina, incontinence or frequent urination, lower back pain and impotency.

Always start with a limited number of repetitions and increase intensity gradually. People with weak internal organs should not practice this type of breathing.

Varying-Length Breathing

By increasing the length of the inhalation or exhalation, or by pausing the breath, different effects are produced. Exhaling longer decreases carbon dioxide, other toxic gas levels, and lowers blood pressure. Exhaling longer also helps you to relax and increases Yin energy.

Inhaling longer helps gather energy, creates more tension, increases blood pressure and Yang energy. Pausing after inhalation builds more Yang Qi while pausing after exhalation builds more Yin Qi.

Light, deep, long, even breathing reaches the cellular level of the body, and is very relaxing. Quick breathing moves the Blood and energizes the body.

Pulsating Breath

Pulsating breath is used to build more Yang Qi or to expel more toxins from the Lungs. For example, the practitioner inhales three times in short breaths followed by one long exhalation to increase Yang Qi. Or the practitioner inhales normally followed by three exhalations in short breaths to expel toxins from the Lungs.

Letting the exhalation vibrate with the rhythm of the Heart fosters deep relaxation and creates high energy levels in the practitioner. Inhale through the nose and exhale with the mouth slightly open, tip of tongue gently placed on the inside of the lower front teeth.

Pronounce the sound **FFUUU** on exhalation and feel the gentle vibration of the heart rhythm on the lips. Exhale longer than you inhale to foster a greater sense of relaxation and strengthen the Heart/Mind connection.

If a person gets dizzy while practicing breathing, he/she is too yang or too yin. There is too little or too much Blood going to the brain. If this happens rest until the dizziness subsides and continue training at a reduced activity level. If the dizziness continues consult your doctor or a medical professional.

Mind Moving Qi

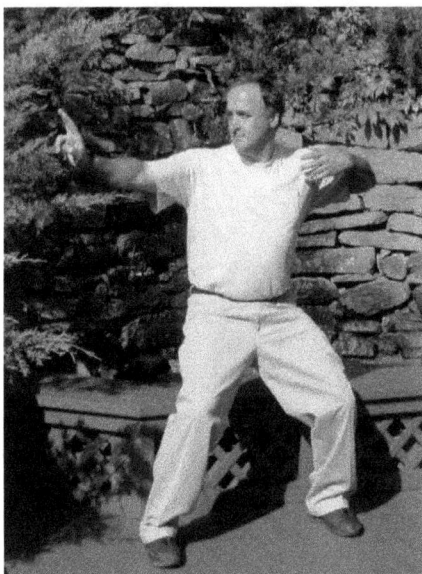

Qi Gong releases ingrained energy patterns that over time may lead to disorder and disease. The power of the Mind helps to release stagnant Qi and bring in clear healthy energy into the body, thus reestablishing a state of balance.

The principle of Mind Moving Qi can be understood as the active mental component of an activity. The idea of intention, Mind intent or Mindfulness implies a level of attention involved in performing an activity.

Energy comes from the Mind to build Qi and improve health. Qi is the vital energy of the body. It is the active motivating force not only of cellular activity, but also of the electromagnetic and subtle energies that circulate in the energy channels of the body.

The Mind directs the vital energy which draws the essence with it. Qi follows whatever the Mind focuses on. The Mind leads the Qi to a certain place. When the Qi is focused there, it gathers essence, and substance will be formed. Physical change will occur.

Imaginal states and the powerful images experienced during these states can produce intense physical experiences that lead to measurable changes in physiological functioning. The creative power of the Mind may manifest in a wide variety of ways, but the essential elements are intent, visualization and conscious awareness.

Webster Dictionary defines intent as the act of turning the Mind toward an object, design or purpose. Ordinarily intent precedes action. We decide on a course of action and follow through with the required steps to achieve our goal. I wish to live a long and healthy life, so I practice Qi Gong every day. My actions follow my intent.

If the purpose of one's intent is to move the Qi in the Microcosmic Orbit, we use the Mind to open the orbit (Governing and Conception Vessels) and visualize the energy moving up the back and down the front of the body in an uninterrupted flow.

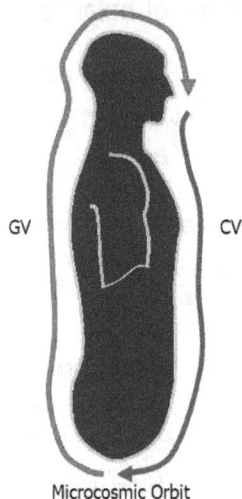

GV

CV

Microcosmic Orbit

In the beginning, we may not necessarily feel the movement of energy in the Microcosmic Orbit. But with disciplined practice and conscious awareness, we begin to sense an opening, and movement in the orbit. The level of practice has evolved from intent, to visualization to conscious awareness of movement of Qi.

The intended action may be to quiet all thoughts and to connect to the flow of universal energy, in other words to let the universal energy direct our actions. This can be called the Mind of no Mind, or the intent of no intent.

Morihei Ueshiba is considered by many as one of Japan's greatest martial artists. He is the founder of the martial art of Aikido, defined as the Way of Blending one's energy with Universal Energy or Ki. The word Ki in Japanese and Qi in Chinese are synonymous.

Ueshiba once reportedly said that to become invincible one must blend with the power of the Universe as no attacker can defeat the Universe. Ueshiba believed that Aikido is the study of the spirit. He constantly urged his students to "link yourself to the Ki of true emptiness."

According to Ueshiba, there are two types of Ki: ordinary Ki and true Ki. Ordinary Ki is coarse and heavy. It creates blockages and stagnates, leading to confusion and maliciousness. True Ki is light and versatile. It creates flowing movement and power. True strength resides where one's Ki is concentrated and stable.

The intent in Qi Gong as in Aikido is to link to the Universal Qi, to be one with the vast emptiness of space or void energy. As Ueshiba once said: "Cast off limiting thoughts and return to true emptiness. Stand in the midst of the Great Void".

Visualization or internal seeing has been defined as the ability to use the "Mind's eye" to see an image and alter it at will. It is the active mental component of an activity.

Visualization is used in many healing arts to effectively harness the power of the Mind. In Qi Gong it is used to release stagnant Qi, build Jing Qi, improve the body's energy flow and connect to the Universal Qi.

Basic to Qi Gong practice is the ability to clear out or to let go of old energy patterns that over time may lead to disease. Visualization is one of the major tools used to dislodge stagnant energy. It also aids in bringing clear energy into the body, thus helping reestablish a state of balance.

In the day-to-day application of visualization, it is helpful to understand the relationship between breath and Qi. Breath and Qi are synonymous. When you move breath, you are moving Qi.

This is demonstrated in many breathing and visualization techniques such as Angle Breathing, Pores Breathing, Sky Sword, Five Element Meditation, Meridian Qi Gong as well as the Micro and Macrocosmic Orbit Meditation.

In some more advanced visualization techniques the relationship between breath and Qi is more difficult to discern. This does not diminish the importance of breath as a support in harnessing the flow of energy in the body. Ultimately the advanced Qi Gong practitioner moves beyond breath to a state of conscious awareness and being.

Ancient Masters

"The ancient Masters were profound and subtle.

Their wisdom was unfathomable.
There is no way to describe it.
All you can describe is their appearance.

They were careful
as someone crossing an iced-over stream.
Alert as a warrior in enemy territory.
Courteous as a guest.
Fluid as melting ice.
Shapeable as a block of wood.
Receptive as a valley.
Clear as a glass of water.

Do you have the patience to wait
till your mud settles and the water is clear?
Can you remain unmoving
till the right action arises by itself?

The Master doesn't seek fulfillment.
Not seeking, not expecting,
he/she is present,
and can welcome all things."

Lao-tzu
Chinese Philosopher

Nine Steps to Mastering Qi Gong

" The Qi Gong student's ability to centre is the basic tool for all energetic practice. Centering is the focused intent that is required to connect with the Universal energy. In addition, the healers physical body needs to be relaxed, the emotions calm, the Mind clear, and the Spirit quiet and still." **Grand Master Shih**

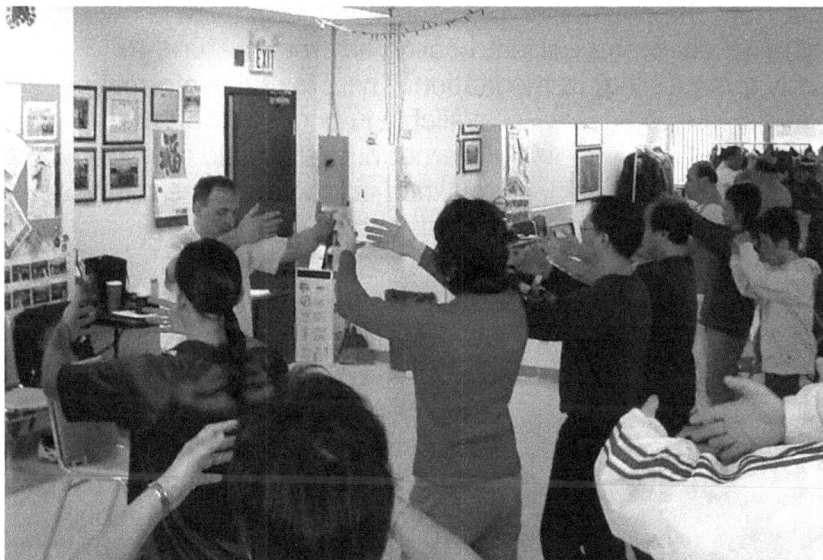

For many the practice of Qi Gong may imply a change of lifestyle. To be healthy sleep at least six hours a night, eat a balanced diet, be physically active, have a positive attitude, and practice Qi Gong every day not only at certain predetermined times of the day but at every opportunity.

Although understanding technique is key to the practice of Qi Gong, the true wisdom of Qi Gong comes from the Heart. During his classes Grandmaster Shih would often repeat: **Smile from the Heart**. This simple exercise brings the Mind under the influence of the Heart's compassion and wisdom, transforming ourselves and our immediate environment. This is positively one of the most powerful and transformative aspects of Qi Gong.

Smiling from the Heart allows one to let go of preconceived ideas and old patterns of behavior to more easily blend with the Qi of the Universe.

To increase one's vitality and strengthen the Jing-Qi-Shen, be part of the Universal Qi, respect its principles, and follow the Nine Steps to Mastering Qi Gong.

1. KNOWLEDGE

To benefit from the practice of Qi Gong, students acquire knowledge about many facets of this ancient healing art from posture, to movement, to breathing, to meditation. There is much information

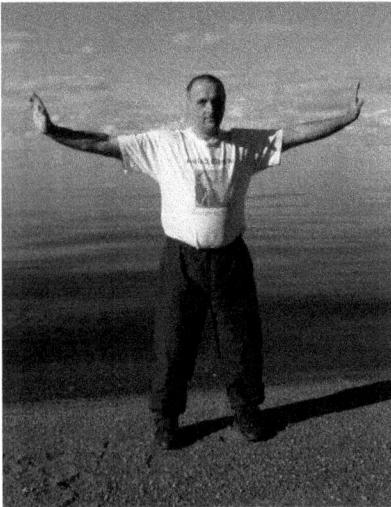

available in books and on the Internet but if possible seek out a qualified instructor. Some things are better learned firsthand by interacting with a Qi Gong instructor.

2. DISCIPLINE

Many students accumulate knowledge about Qi Gong but never succeed in practicing on a regular basis. The accumulation of knowledge seems to become the sole objective. A certain comfort is gotten from this, but true knowledge comes from experience and experience comes only from regular and sustained practice.

3. REGULATE THE BODY

Relaxing the body is the first step in the practice of Qi Gong. To relax the body, first adopt proper posture. It helps reduce resistance to the circulation of Qi, enables you to better focus the Mind, and opens the body to Universal Energy. Posture reflects the state of the Mind. Proper posture helps bring your Mind and body to centre and enables you to move with awareness and fluidity.

4. REGULATE BREATH

The breath should be soft, slow, silent and deep. This enables you to relax in a more Mindful and effective practice. The breath reflects the state of the Qi and the Mind. Use it to delve deeper into your essential being. Experienced practitioners breathe at a rhythm of 2 to 5 breaths per minute.

5. REGULATE THE MIND

A tranquil Mind makes the body relaxed and supple, increasing Qi flow. Let the eyebrows drop and mouth relax. Yin Tang (Mid-eyebrow point) opens and this connects the Heart and brain. **Smile from the heart.** It helps avoid buildup of stagnant or rebellious Qi.

6. REGULATE THE SPIRIT

We are like grains of sand in a vast Universe. The energy around us is immense. Be **open with the Universe, keep the Spirit up** and you will never deplete your own Qi or be exhausted by the stress of daily life.

7. DEVELOP GOOD CHARACTER

The way we think impacts the quality of our Qi. Acquired Qi is influenced by how we live and by our emotions. Harbor no desires and have good thoughts, develop a good Mind to keep the Qi in the body. Think in a way that helps you harmonize with the natural environment.

We lose Qi if we are angry, sad, jealous, fearful, too happy or too excited, if we think too much or worry or show a lack of confidence in ourselves and others. We need lots of love, a Heart that can receive everything. Spend time on what makes you happy. The practice of Qi Gong helps balance emotions.

8. NO HURRY

Avoid looking to the future. Live in the present moment. This brings you into focus and increases your level of sensitivity and energy.

9. NO WORRY

Worry is fear of the future. It leads to guilt, negativity and loss of self-empowerment, and eventually to loss of health. Do not be scared or rebellious Qi will weaken you.

How to Maximize Practice

"Daily training in the Art of Peace allows your inner divinity to shine brighter and brighter. Do not concern yourself with the right or wrong of others. Do not be calculating or act unnatural. Keep your Mind set on the Art of Peace, and do not criticize other teachers or traditions. The art of Peace never restrains, restricts, or shackles anything. It embraces all and purifies everything." **Morihei Ueshiba, Founder of Aikido**

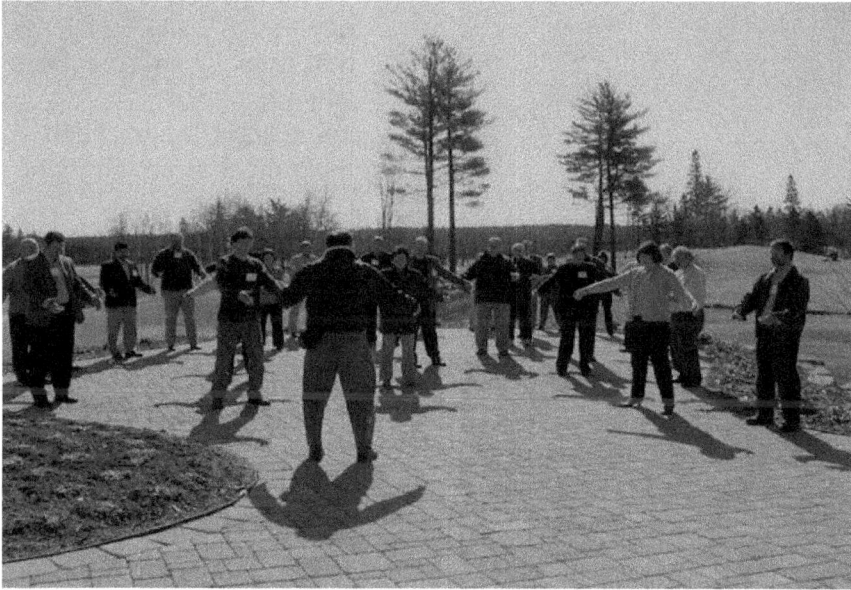

The more you practice the more Qi you will cultivate. Do not expect immediate results. Changes brought about by the regular practice of Qi Gong can be immediate but are more often subtle. Appreciate the positive results Qi Gong brings to your health and well-being. This will motivate you to continue practice.

To be successful do not be goal oriented. How you practice makes a big difference. Focus on enjoying the journey and not on reaching the destination.

You also need knowledge of proper technique and the ability to remain tranquil. Practicing **relax, no hurry, no worry,** creates the appropriate condition to increase Qi and promote its abundant circulation.

The best time to practice Qi Gong is at dawn before breakfast. Drink a glass of water before the start of practice. Qi moves more easily in the meridians when the body is hydrated. This also helps improve peristalsis. Remove jewelry and wear loose, comfortable clothing. Practice in a peaceful and well-ventilated location.

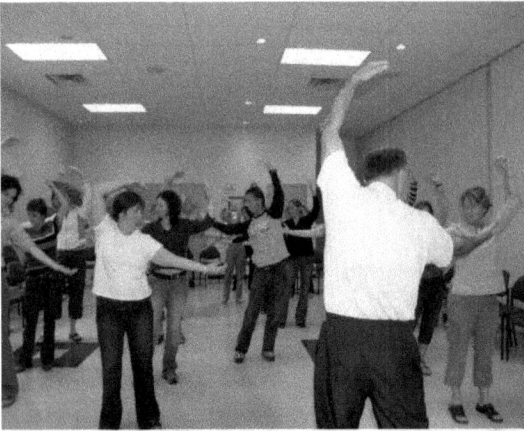

It is good to practice in the same location every day as you build up Qi in that area. Do not practice when hungry or immediately after eating a big meal as the Qi cultivated through practice will be directed towards the digestive process instead of building up your vital energy.

When you practice Qi Gong the pores of the body open. So to avoid getting a cold do not practice in the rain. The back and spine have a lot of points that are connected to the internal organs. So avoid wind on the back.

Moderate wind from the front is fine as it is not easy to catch cold. Moderate wind to the head is also fine as it moves from the head down the outside of the arms and massages the body. The feet are doors to the earth, so it is easy to catch cold through the feet.

Do not practice Qi Gong in thunder and lightning as it may interfere with the movement of energy in the body. If the demands of everyday life do not permit you to complete your regular practice, focus on one or two exercises that you can complete in a short period of time. Remain relaxed and do not hurry. A short-focused practice helps maintain your progress in Qi Gong.

When practicing Qi Gong, it is important to smile from the heart. Your feet are rooted to the earth. Imagine the crown of the head suspended from above. The movements are soft, continuous and effortless. Always stay within your natural ability.

The Mind and Heart work together to strengthen the body. We need a lot of love, a Heart that can receive everything. Work on character and emotions to have stronger Qi. If our emotions are unbalanced for too long, it weakens Qi.

The value of Qi Gong is in lasting practice with an empty Mind, natural breathing, and harmony of energy and breath. Over time, Qi Gong becomes a way of life. Regular practice leads to improved posture, better balance, and deeper more relaxed breathing.

Improved posture and balance help move the Blood and Qi in the body. Belly breathing improves concentration and helps reduce the stress of everyday life. Smiling from the heart transforms our reactions to negative emotions and difficult events. You become the person you were destined to be and can positively influence those around you simply by the way you are.

To achieve this, think about things that help us harmonize and fit into the natural environment. Help people be beautiful and better morally. This gives us greater wisdom.

Getting Rid of Toxic Energy

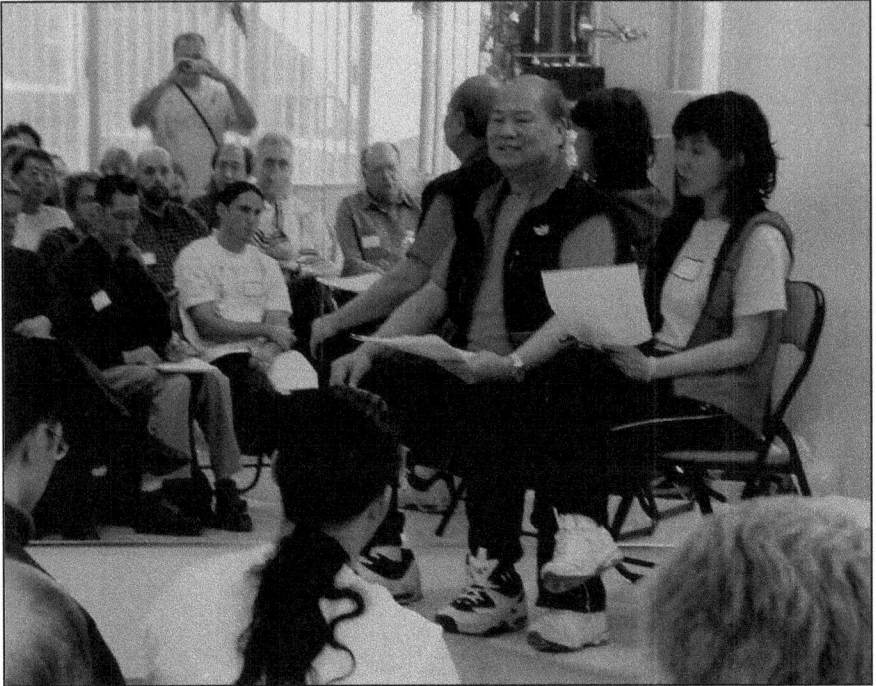

A few years before he died Master Weizhao Wu gathered together friends of Qi Gong and many of his students to talk about the importance of virtue in the practice of Qi Gong. I was fortunate to have been able to travel to Toronto, Ontario, Canada, to attend this presentation. I will endeavor to summarize his talk.

When practicing Qi Gong the terms "negative and sad energy" are often used to better describe the effects of various types of Qi. In fact, energy cannot be negative, bad or sad. In technical terms, it can be described as toxic, overflowing, stagnant, deficient, balanced or rebellious.

We perceive people with balanced energy as happy, positive and vibrant. We perceive people with stagnant or rebellious energy as sad or negative. Using descriptive terms helps better understand how energy works.

In his presentation Master Wu indicated that above all remember the importance of virtue. Be kind. Cultivate a good Mind. Fear, anger or desire depletes your energy. Smile with everything, be happy with everything, enjoy life and cultivate energy. The body energy needs to circulate. If there is too much tension the energy doors will close. You need to be happy for energy to come.

A happy Mind is open. Sad energy goes out and down. Fear energy dissipates. Tension, worry energy tightens. There is no need to worry, to hurry or to get angry. Be happy, relaxed and peaceful. This balances the energy in the whole body. With a correct Mind and Spirit, the body will be healthier.

Toxic Qi can come from external sources. We do not know when toxic Qi will enter the body. A weakened immune system, external injuries or negative influences can cause blockages allowing external pathogens to invade the body.

It is important to practice Qi Gong to strengthen resistance to disease and allow Qi to pass through the energy blockages. There is therefore less chance of being sick, less chance toxic Qi will enter the body.

Extreme emotions can throw us off track especially if we remain unbalanced for a long period of time. The way we think has an impact on our emotions. We lose Qi if we are angry, jealous, or have a lack of confidence in others or ourselves. If we worry or are afraid we lose Qi.

Work on our character and emotions to have better Qi. A little smile on the face works magic. Let the eyebrows drop and jaw relax. The Yin Tang (mid-eyebrow point) opens and this connects the Heart and the brain creating a greater sense of harmony within yourself and with others.

There are many reasons to be angry. Do not get so angry so it comes from the Heart. Extreme emotions – too angry, too happy, and too sad - weaken Qi. Above all control anger. The way the Mind and Heart work together impacts on Qi. If our emotions upset us for a long period of time, it weakens the Qi.

If your Mind is not happy, it creates tension. Many energy gates or doors close. Tension starts when we are born when we cry for food and love. As we get older we think too much. We get caught up in jealousy and competition. Be happy with other people's success.

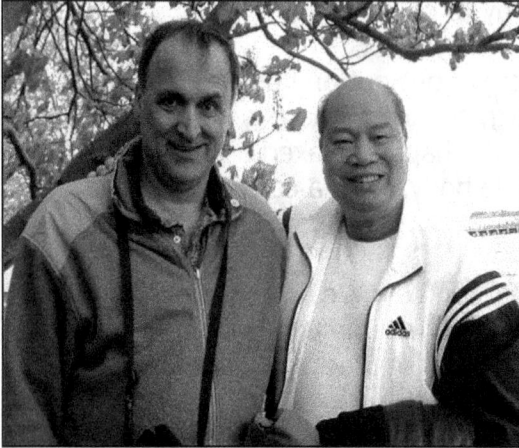

Understand that we are complete. Be always happy and your energy will always be open. Even if someone is mad at you, you are still happy. Believe in yourself and you will do good for society. Keep your Mind always happy and your energy will always be balanced and circulate freely and abundantly.

The following are additional tips on how to avoid getting drained by toxic energy.

- Be Positive

The way we think impacts character. Think in a way that helps us harmonize and fit into our natural environment. We must want to do well, help people be beautiful and respect everyone's beliefs.

Sometimes we live in extremes, so we become off track with our emotions. Do not hate others or desire what they have.

- Be Grounded

Adopt proper posture. Bring your Mind and body to the one-point located in the center of the lower abdomen.

- Practice Soft Breathing

Develop a quiet, slow, deep and tranquil breath.

60

- Cultivate a Tranquil Mind

Relax the eyebrows. Smile from the heart. A tranquil Mind makes the body relaxed and supple, increasing Qi flow.

- Be Opened with the Universe

Use the Mind to make the whole body as big as the Universe. Maintain a sense of openness with the Universe in everything you do.

- Practice Self-Healing Qi Gong

Practice Qi Gong to develop strong Qi and strengthen the weaker parts of the body.

External Qi healers must practice self-healing Qi Gong to stay in an optimal, fully charged energy state. Regular Qi Gong practice makes you a more sensitive and effective healer, and helps you avoid losing your personal energy.

Pathogenic Factors

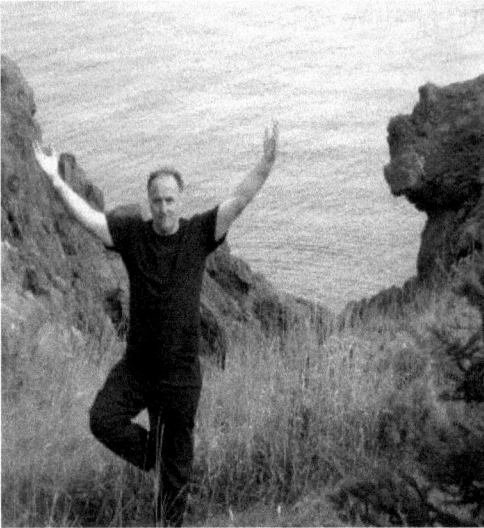

In Traditional Chinese Medicine (TCM) the Heart governs the Blood vessels. A happy and calm Heart keeps the Mind clear. The Spleen controls the Blood. It transforms energy from food and sends it to the Lungs. The Lungs transform Qi from the air which floats down like mist to the Kidneys. The Kidneys house the Jing or Essential Qi. They provide the bone marrow that nourishes the Brain. The Liver circulates Qi and harmonizes the emotions.

The main pathology of the Heart is Heat and Inflammation. The Spleen is Dampness, the Lungs is Dryness, the Kidneys Cold and Pain and the Liver Wind conditions, which often lead to joint or muscle pain that comes and goes or moves from place to place.

In TCM disease arises from one or a combination of Six External Evils, Seven Internal Factors, and Eight Miscellaneous Factors. The Six External Evils or Pathogenic Factors arise from the following climatic changes: Wind, Summer Heat, Dampness, Dryness, Cold and Fire.

The Seven Internal Factors arise from excessive internal emotions such as anger, joy, worry, grief, sadness, fear and shock.

The Eight Miscellaneous causes of disease are overexertion, diet, trauma, constitutional factors, excessive sex, frequent child bearing, exposure to poisons or parasites, and iatrogenic disorders (consequence of medical treatment or advice).

When a patient arrives at a TCM clinic, a variety of methods are used to collect the information on signs and symptoms needed to identify the pattern of disharmony that is at the root of a disorder. A TCM practitioner looks at the physical, emotional, environmental and spiritual aspects of the patient.

Questioning, visual observation, listening, smelling, palpation, tongue and pulse diagnosis are the major tools used to establish a list of signs and symptoms. A pattern of disharmony is then identified using many diagnostic methods such as:

- The Eight Principles (Yin, Yang / Excess, Deficient / Internal, External / Hot, Cold)

- The identification of Qi, Blood and Body Fluids

- The Four Levels or Stages of Heat (Wei Qi or Protective Level, Qi Level, Ying or Nutritive Level, and Xue or Blood Level)

- The Six Stages of Penetration of Cold (Greater Yang, Brighter Yang, Lesser Yang, Greater Yin, Lesser Yin and Terminal Yin)

- The Emotional Factors

- The Major Organ Patterns

- The Five Elements Theory (Fire, Earth, Metal, Water and Wood)

In addition, practitioners of Qi Gong and other forms of energy medicine often rely on Intuitive and Perceptual Diagnosis to identify the root cause of disease.

The practice of Qi Gong not only improves overall health and longevity, it also sharpens the intuitive and perceptual abilities of the practitioner. But like in any discipline, it is important to master the basics to fully benefit from the hours of practice required to truly understand the essence of the art.

The Five Element Theory

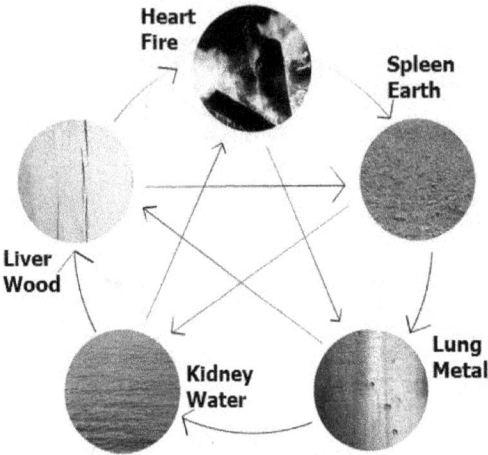

The Five Element Theory was developed by the ancient Chinese Physicians to help understand the connections between the physiology and pathology of the organs and tissues, and the natural environment. According to this theory, Wood, Fire, Earth, Metal, and Water are the basic elements of the material world. Wood represents the Liver, Fire the Heart, Earth the Spleen, Metal the Lungs, and Water the Kidneys.

These elements are in constant movement and change. The complex connections between material objects are explained through the relationship of interdependence and mutual restraint that governs the five elements. For example, Wood, which represents the Liver, supports Fire which represents the Heart, but controls Earth which represents the Spleen. Fire, which represents the Heart, supports Earth which represents the Spleen, but controls Metal which represents the Lungs.

The two relationships mentioned above are the Supporting and the Controlling relationships. Together they foster balance and harmony in the system. Each element supports the next one in the cycle and each element controls another, keeping all elements and organs systems in balance.

The following chart describes a few of the indicators associated with the Five Elements such as the corresponding Organ, Color, Virtues, Acquired Emotions, and related Tissue.

Organ	Element & Color	Basic Virtue	Acquired Emotions	Tissue
Heart/ Small Intestine	Fire Red	**Order** = Peace & Boundary Setting, Love, Forgiveness, Joy, Happiness	Shock, Fright Nervousness Excitement	Blood Vessels

Organ	Element & Color	Basic Virtue	Acquired Emotions	Tissue
Spleen/ Stomach	Earth Yellow	**Trust** = Faith, Honesty, Openness, Acceptance, Truthfulness, Peace of Mind, Meditation, Contemplation	Worry, Remorse, Regret, Self-Doubt, Obsessiveness Pensiveness, Over-thinking	Flesh/ Muscles

Organ	Element & Color	Basic Virtue	Acquired Emotions	Tissue
Lung/ Large Intestine	Metal White	**Integrity** = Righteousness, Dignity, Social Responsibility	Sadness, Sorrow, Worry Grief, Guilt Shame, Anxiety, Disappointment	Skin/ Body Hair

Organ	Element & Color	Basic Virtue	Acquired Emotions	Tissue
Kidney/ Bladder	Water Mid-night Blue or Black	**Wisdom** = Rational Mind, Clear Perception, Self-Understanding	Fear, Extreme Anxiety, Loneliness, Insecurity	Bones/ Brain Marrow

Organ	Element & Color	Basic Virtue	Acquired Emotions	Tissue
Liver/ Gall Bladder	Wood Green	**Kindness** = Benevolence, Compassion, Assertiveness	Anger, Irritability, Blame, Resentment, Rage, Frustration, Bitterness, Moodiness, Jealousy, Depression	Sinews/ Tendons

In many instances, the Five Element Theory has a direct application to the practice of Qi Gong. For example, exercises that strengthen the Kidney Water help cool the Heart Fire and strengthen the Liver Wood. This is based on the observation that Water extinguishes Fire while nourishing the growth of trees or Wood.

Excessive emotions such as fear will weaken the Kidneys. Therefore, cultivating a sense of tranquility in the face of fear will strengthen the Kidneys enabling you to better react to a perceived threat.

The main pathology associated with the Kidneys is arthritis which can be interpreted as the fear of moving forward in life to fulfill one's destiny. Healthy Kidneys maintain a strong life force which helps prevent the occurrence of this disorder.

The Spleen has influence over muscles. Worry and regret weaken the Spleen and may lead overtime to reduced muscle tone especially in the upper limbs.

We exercise the external body by strengthening and stretching the muscles. But we often forget the importance the internal organs play in maintaining a high level of health and happiness.

In Qi Gong, various methods are used to strengthen the organ systems such as developing basic virtues, meditating on the color of the Yin organs, pronouncing the organ's healing sound, and using the Mind to move the Qi in the organ meridian network. Body movement is also incorporated into the mix to stretch the meridian pathways and compress the targeted organ.

Both the Mind and the body are called upon to focus the healing power of Qi onto the major organ systems often with very positive results.

Healing Sounds

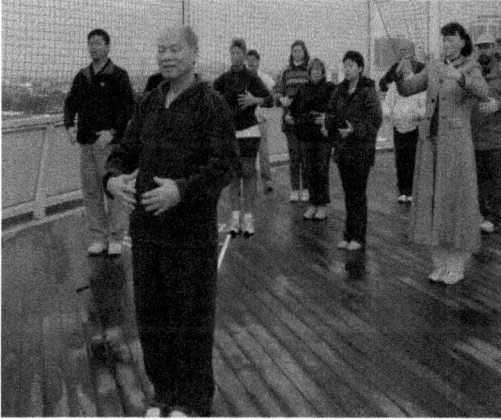

Healing sounds or words occupy a dominant role in helping release stagnant Qi in the organ systems thus facilitating the flow of energy in the major organs and meridians. The use of sound in the martial and healing arts has a long history. During the Sui Dynasty (590 - 618 A.D.), a Taintai Buddhist high priest, Zhi Zhuan, pointed out the healing potential of the Six Healing Sounds or Words. The Six Healing Sounds were first recorded as *Chui, Hu, Xi, Ke, Xu, and Si.*

All matter vibrates at specific frequencies. These frequencies correspond to different colors and different sounds. Pronouncing a sound that matches the frequency of a specific part of the body helps release deep-rooted tension. Release of tension brings more energy and Blood to the area thus improving health.

Several Qi Gong exercises use shaking of the body to release stagnant Qi. The shaking movement can be subtle as in Dancing with the Universe, a style that promotes spontaneous movement. Or it can be more obvious as in the Shaking or Dropping of Posts exercises.

Shaking, much like the vibrations created by sound, facilitate the release of deep rooted tension in the muscles, joints and connective tissue.

Each of the major organs - Lungs, Spleen, Heart, Kidneys, Liver and the Triple Warmer - vibrates at a specific energy frequency. Each of the Six Healing Sounds match specific organ frequencies to help target the healing power of Qi.

Healing Sounds can also be used to open and relax the whole body down to the cellular level. This helps further condense Universal Qi into the body. **SOONG,** which means relax in Chinese, is often used in Qi Gong opening and closing exercises to help let go of deep-rooted tension. **FFUUU,** which means to open, is used to harmonize the breath with the heart rhythm further relaxing the body. Another sound used to help release tension and consolidate the Qi is **AAHHH.**

Pronouncing the sound of the Zang or Yin organs plus the Triple Warmer promotes their overall health, harmonizes the relationship between them, and clears any existing energetic imbalances. This type of meditation is based on the theory of the Five Elements.

The following is an interpretation of the six healing sounds and colors that I believe best reflect the energy vibrations of the targeted organs. Also include are descriptions of the movement of Qi in the related meridians.

Please note that the Qi in the Yin meridians of the arms moves away from the center of the body to the extremities while the Qi in the Yin meridians of the legs move from the extremities towards the center of the body.

The Triple Warmer is a Yang Organ. Its Qi moves from the extremities towards the center of the body.

Zang or Yin Organs	Healing Sounds	Organ Opening & Color	Moving Qi in Meridians
Liver	"Shu...e...e...e" The tongue is cupped and loosely touching the upper teeth. The lower lip is farther out. Smile, with the center of the lips together. The sound moves out the corner of the lips to the eyes vibrating both the sides of the mouth and the Liver. Keep the eyes wide open.	Eyes/ Green	Move the Qi up the lateral side of the big toe to the inside of the leg and groin, up to the floating rib, moving internally up to the sides of the mouth, eyes and brain.

Heart	"Haw...w...w...w" With the mouth open wide and rounded, place the tip of the tongue lightly on the inside of the lower teeth. Vibrate both the tongue and the Heart.	Tongue/ Red	Move the Qi from the armpit down the inside of the arm and forearm to inside of the little finger.
Spleen	"Huu...u...u" Pronounced "Whooooo". The lips are rounded. The jaw is slightly open and the tongue curled slightly downward. Vibrate both the inside of the mouth and the Spleen.	Mouth/ Yellow	Move the Qi from the inside of the big toe up the inside of the legs up to the groin to the outside of the ribs to below the collar bone, and then down six finger widths to the area under the armpit.
Lung	"See...e...e" With the mouth slightly open, upper and lower teeth opposite each other, lightly press the tip of the tongue against the lower teeth, so the air can exit through the opening while pronouncing the healing sound. Vibrate both the nose and the Lungs.	Nose/ White	Move the Qi from the front sides of the chest near the armpit down the inside of the arm to the inside of the elbow down the forearm to the inside of the thumb.
Kidney	"Chwa...a...a...y" Place the tongue as far back in the mouth as possible like a sail pointing towards the roof of the mouth. Widen the corners of the mouth. The sound vibrates both the ears and the Kidneys.	Ears/ Mid- night Blue or Black	Move the Qi from the center of the foot up the inside of the leg to the groin, and then to the medial end of the collar bone.
Triple Burner	"She...e...e" Place the tip of the tongue on the lower teeth. Vibrate the whole tongue as it represents all the organs as well as the Triple Warmer, which extends from the base of the tongue to the pelvic floor. The air travels over the entire tongue. The mouth is slightly open so the air can escape more easily.	Tongue Orange Red	Move the Qi from the outside of the ring finger up the outside of the hand, forearm and arm, to the Great Vertebrae, around the back of the ear, to the outside of the eyebrow.

Different forms of meditation are used to strengthen the energy of the organs. The first method uses a ball of fire to heat the targeted organ and intensify its natural color.

Sit comfortably on the edge of a chair. Once you achieve a state of inner quiet, imagine a ball of fire hovering at the mid-eyebrow point or Yin Tang. After a few moments, let the ball of fire enter the Yin Tang and move to the pineal gland located at the center of the head. Then let the fireball drop to the targeted organ.

As the organ heats up it creates more energy and more color. For example, imagine the ball of fire entering the Yin Tang, moving to the pineal gland, and dropping down to the Heart. As the Heart gets warmer, its red color intensifies. Hold this visualization for a few moments before moving to another organ.

When practicing this style, follow the supporting organ sequence starting with the Heart, followed by the Spleen, Lungs, Kidneys and Liver. After completing the sequence rest the Mind in the Lower Dantian. See the diagram on page 64.

Another method combines the color of the organ with its healing sound. Once you achieve a state of inner quiet, inhale while focusing on the healthy and vibrant color of the targeted organ. Exhale pronouncing the organ's healing sound vibrating both the targeted organ and its opening to the exterior.

The Kidneys open to the ears, the Heart to the tongue, the Lungs to the nose, the Liver to the eyes, and the Spleen to the mouth. As in the first method, follow the supporting organ sequence starting with the Heart, followed by the Spleen, Lungs, Kidneys and Liver. After completing the sequence rest the Mind in the Lower Dantian.

The final version adds body movement to the mix as well as the movement of Qi in the related meridian system. This method is explained in my third book on Qi Gong entitled Dance of the Dragon - Healing Oneself & Others.

Acupressure Self-Help

Acupressure or the application of pressure with the hands or feet to specific points on the body is an important part of Traditional Chinese Medicine, and Qi Gong. Acupuncture and acupressure use the same points to stimulate the body's self-curative abilities.

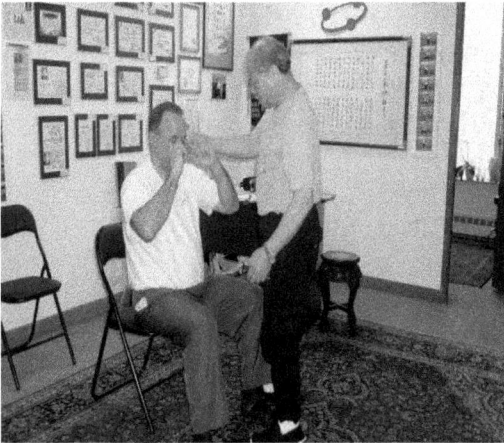

The use of acupressure supports the practice of Qi Gong by releasing stagnant Qi strengthening the body's immune system. Acupressure helps increase energy levels, balance the flow of energy, reduce pain and improve overall health. It also lowers tension and stress providing a greater sense of harmony, health and well-being.

Acupressure points are located on both sides of the body except for the points located on the Conception Vessel and Governing Vessel, which are found on the center line of the body. The points are usually massaged by rotating the thumb or fingers ten to twelve times on the point and applying firm pressure for 30 seconds.

The palms can be used to massage the face and neck as well as the abdomen and sides of the body. The heels of the feet can be used to rub the tops of the feet and lateral sides of the lower legs.

When held for an extended period, various Yoga poses are also effective in activating acupressure points. When lying on the back, the weight of the body on the practice mat applies pressure to important spinal and bladder points located along the spine. A half headstand applies pressure on scalp points important for achieving motor-sensory balance.

The reclining spinal twist applies pressure on bladder and gallbladder points in the buttocks, helpful in relieving hip and sciatic pain, while the Sphinx and Cobra apply pressure to Liver and Kidney points along lower abdomen.

The Qi Gong styles presented in this book as well as in my second book entitled, Qi Gong's Five Golden Keys, activate several acupressure points such as the Window of the Sky Point located in the depression just above the sternum, used to help relieve respiratory distress, and the Lumbar Eyes located on the lower back about 3 to 4 inches lateral to each side of the 4th lumbar vertebrae, used to strengthen the Kidneys and release lower back tension.

Tapping, rubbing and stretching also helps activate acupoints and stimulate stagnant areas of the body. Drumming the occipital protuberance located on the back of the head opens Bladder and Gall Bladder points that benefit the ears and eyes and helps the Qi move more freely in the Micro Cosmic Orbit.

Flexing and extending the hips opens the Gate of Life and Sea of Qi points strengthening the lumbar spine and fortifying Yang Qi.

Rubbing the sides of the ears activates points along the Gall Bladder, Triple Warmer and Small Intestine Meridians, clearing the head and benefiting the ears.

Many Qi Gong styles end with a facial, neck and scalp massage that help beautify facial skin, relieve pain and open congested areas.

Energy Enhancing Food

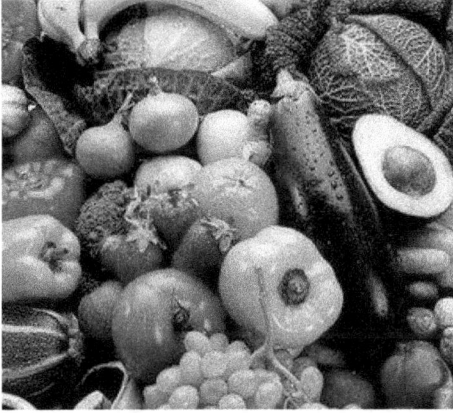

Approximately 35% of your energy is spent every day in the process of digestion and elimination. To be healthy eat a balanced diet. Avoid processed foods. Limit consumption of saturated fats, salt and sugar. Eat lots of fresh fruits and vegetables.

Foods generally fall into three categories: proteins, carbohydrates and fats. Proteins from red meat are the most difficult for the body to break down and require the longest time to process. Therefore, these proteins are ideally eaten during the morning or before mid-afternoon.

Certain proteins are less stressful for the body to assimilate. Low-stress proteins provide more energy than they consume. Some examples of this are sprouted beans, chicken, coconut, cottage cheese, nuts soaked in water, ocean fish, scallops, soy ferments, tofu and wild rice.

Acid forming foods also drain energy from the body. It is more difficult for illness to manifest in a body that is more alkaline. To avoid stressing the body avoid excessive consumption of acid forming foods such as eggs, dairy products, meat, fish, most grains, alcohol and soft drinks, white sugar, artificial sweeteners, coffee, condiments, black tea, chocolate, yeast products, as well as processed, fermented and refined foods.

Balance off the acidic nature of these foods with regular consumption of vegetables, which should be the focus of your diet, plus fruits, fresh grains that are slightly acidic such as amaranth, quinoa and spelt, fresh grains that are between neutral and slightly alkaline such as millet and buckwheat, as well as sea vegetables, chestnuts, natural sugar such as honey, cold-pressed oils, and sprouts.

In China food is classified according to easily observed patterns. People who feel overheated should eat cooling foods while people who feel cold should eat warming foods. Detoxifying foods are for those who carry excess toxins. Building foods are good for deficient persons.

Building foods nourish the Blood. The best foods to build and nourish Blood are from plant sources and include dark green leafy vegetables, seaweeds, spirulina, sprouts, legumes and whole grains.

Richly colored foods (often red) are valued for building the Blood including goji berries (Chinese wolf berries), dried apricots, dark grapes, blackberries, raspberries and black strap molasses.

In addition, animal sources such as organic meat, eggs and Liver, and soups based on meat bone broth nourish blood but should be used in limited quantities.

According to LotusRootAcupuncture.com, **bitter foods** such as rhubarb and dandelion leaf tend to descend the Qi, drain heat and dry dampness. Some bitter foods have a purgative effect as they induce bowel movements. Energetically, the flavor bitter affects the Heart and the Spirit (Shen). Bitter foods eaten in excess injure the bones.

Sour foods such as grapefruit and olives are astringent, cooling and generate Yin fluids. In small amounts, they aid digestion. Energetically, the flavor sour goes to the Liver and Spirit Soul (Hun). Sour foods eaten in excess injure the nerves.

Pungent or spicy foods such as ginger and cayenne pepper have a warming action, promoting energy to move upwards and outwards to the body's surface, moving Qi and circulating the Blood. They also are useful to disperse mucus from the Lungs. Energetically, the flavor spicy goes to the Lungs and animal Soul (Po). Pungent foods eaten in excess injure the Qi.

Salty foods such as kelp and soya sauce are cooling and hold fluids in the body. They have a downward flowing action, soften hardness and act as a purgative. Energetically, the flavor salty goes to the Kidney which houses the spirit of will, determination and drive (Zhi). Salty foods eaten in excess injure the Blood.

Sweet foods can be divided into two groups:

1) Sweet foods that are neutral and nourishing, or warm and nourishing. These include meat, legumes, nuts, dairy products and starchy vegetables

2) Sweet foods that are cooling. These include fruits, sugar, honey and other sweeteners, as well as potatoes, rice and apples. Energetically, the flavor sweet is tonifying and goes to the Spleen and Mind (Yi). Sweet foods eaten in excess injure the muscles.

According to Paul Pitchford, author of Healing with Whole Foods, Asian Traditions and Modern Nutrition, "when a good attitude and sufficient exercise are combined with a balanced diet, there is no limit to health. Emphasize not food but the Essence within every aspect of reality, including food."

A brief period of stillness before a meal as well as eating in a peaceful setting helps with digestion and assimilation of nutrients.

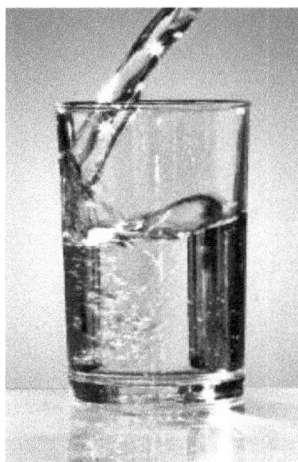

Next to air, water is the most essential element to our survival. Our cells live in an aquatic environment. They swim in an ocean of liquid and are both surrounded and filled with water.

The body should therefore always be well hydrated, so the cells and enzymes have enough water to function properly.

Digestion, assimilation, growth, tissue repair, elimination, energy production, and more all depend on the healthy activity of cells and enzymes. It is no wonder that water plays a key role in the prevention of disease.

Whereas too much water can cause coldness, weaken digestion and deplete the body's energy, insufficient water consumption can lead to accumulation of toxins in the body, constipation, dryness, tension, inflammation, overeating, and Kidney damage.

The most important principle regarding personal water consumption is listening to the wisdom of one's own body and drinking according to thirst.

Since water is such an important component to our health, it would make sense that the quality of the water is also important. Good quality water is clean and free of contaminants and possess a balanced pH or acid-alkaline level. Drinking healthy water helps balance the body's pH and facilitates the elimination of acid waste lodged deep in body tissue.

Dragon Qi Gong

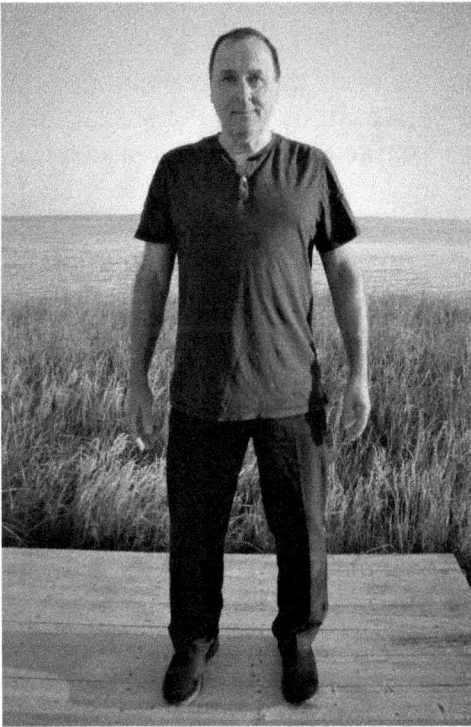

Dragon Qi Gong is an introductory style of Qi Gong that promotes health and longevity. As always, remember the key points when practicing Qi Gong. (Refer to Body Posture)

- Feet rooted to the earth
- Crown of head suspended from above
- Keep the movements soft, continuous and effortless
- Open the body to the Universe
- Smile from the Heart
- Relax: No Hurry, No Worry
- Be peaceful inside and humble outside
- In doing the exercises, stay within your natural ability

First adopt a standing posture with the following indications:

- Feet shoulder width apart, 70% of body weight on the heels, knees straight but soft, abdomen pressed gently against the lower back, chin in with Adam's apple raised slightly upward.

- Arms hang down the sides of the body with palms of hands open and facing the sides of the body.

- Anus is closed and the tip of tongue gently placed on the upper palate behind the front teeth.

- Align the three points: Crown of Head, Center of the Perineum, and the Midpoint of the line connecting the heels of the feet.

- Practice with soft eyes that are fully open, or half closed looking to the horizon.

1. Shifting Weight to Release Tension

Reconnect with the earth and unwind tensions by letting the body weight shift from front to back, and back to front. Feel the shift from the balls of the feet to the heels and from the heels to the balls of the feet.

Let the body relax and unwind, moving in a gentle wave from front to back and back to front letting go of tension. After a few minutes let the body move to a still point with its weight 70% on the heels. Relax in the Wu Ji posture. (Posture of limitless void)

2. Relaxation with SOONG

The word SOONG means relaxation of the Mind, of the spirit and of the body. It implies quietness, softness, flexibility, sinking, openness and emptiness as well as being free of obstructions.

Relax each part of the body making the sound SOONG when exhaling. Relax the head, neck, shoulders, chest, abdomen, upper back, lower back, arms/hands and fingers, hips and groin area, legs/feet and toes. Repeat from 3 to 6 times. Then relax the whole body from head to toes 3 to 6 times.

When you inhale, use the Mind to open the part of the body you are focusing on as big as the Universe. When you exhale, pronounce the healing sound SOONG. When pronouncing the word SOONG, let the nose vibrate with the healing sound as well as the part of the body you are focusing on.

3. Belly Breathing to Open the Lower and Middle Dantian

Relaxed Belly Breathing is practiced throughout most of the form, except when an alternate form of breathing is required, as it helps relax both the Mind and the body making the practice more effective.

Inhale through the nose, to the count of seven, expanding the lower part of the body, front, side and back. Exhale through the nose to the count of ten letting the chest drop down. Repeat 10 to 30 times. The breath is gentle, silent, slow, deep and unbroken. Let the inhalation rise on its own from the space between exhalation and inhalation. Thirty breaths equal approximately five minutes.

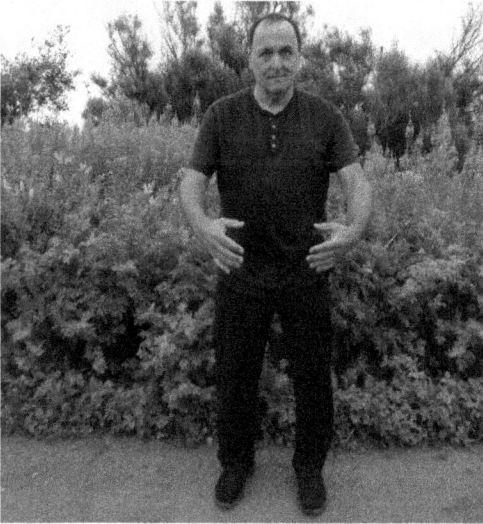

Move the hands to the front of the body, as shown in the picture, palms facing the lower Dantian about two fists away from the abdomen. As you inhale, let the hands expand outward from the lower Dantian about the width of two fists. As you exhale, let the hands move back to the original position. Imagine an energetic connection between the palm centers and the center of the Lower Dantian. Repeat for 10 breaths.

Raise the arms to shoulder height facing the Middle Dantian and continue Relaxed Belly Breathing. The arms are immobile but soft, like they are floating effortlessly in the air.

As you inhale move the hands away from the body about the width of two fists letting the middle of the chest gently open. As you exhale, let the hands and mid chest area move back to the original position. Imagine an energetic connection between the palm centers and the center of the Middle Dantian. Repeat for 10 breaths.

4. Bringing Down the Heavens

Inhale and arch back, arms reaching up towards the sky, palms facing upward, chin in, head and chest facing in the same direction, gently tightening the abdomen.

Gather universal Qi from the stars, galaxies, and empty space. Exhale, and straighten the body. The palms are now hovering above the Crown of the head. Let the universal energy flow down over the whole body.

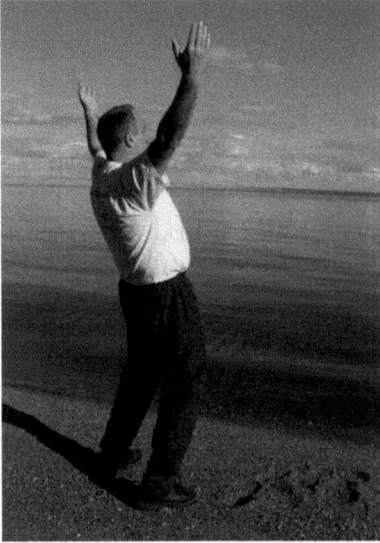

Shift the body weight from front to back and back to front letting the body move in a wave like motion for about 6 to 9 repetitions. The movement starts at the feet and moves gently upward to the tips of the fingers in a wave-like motion.

After about 6 repetitions still the body. Then as you exhale let the palms move down the front of the body bringing the Universal energy down to the Lower Dantian.

Once you reach full extension of the arms at the hips, let the palms move to the sides of the body, using the Mind to release stagnant Qi deep into the earth.

Then as you inhale raise the arms up the sides of the body. About halfway up rotate the forearms so the palms are facing the sky. Arch back once again arms reaching up towards the sky and repeat the movement as before. Repeat 6 to 9 times.

5. Turtle Qi Gong

Turtle Qi Gong consists of rotations of the cervical spine left and right while Eating Air and Swallowing Saliva or the **Pill of Immortality**.

The ancients in China believed that by eating air one could live for long periods without the need for food. Air contains nitrogen, hydrogen, carbon and oxygen, which can be transformed into protein and carbohydrates in the body.

The ancients also believed that saliva or the Pill of Immortality contains special antiseptic properties that help kill germs in the digestive track. It improves digestion and strengthens peristalsis.

It relaxes the Stomach and Liver and can help you lose weight without losing energy. Swallowing the Pill of Immortality also helps strengthen the Jing Qi or essence located in the Lower Dantian. This exercise is best practiced in a peaceful place with fresh air and trees, which provide more oxygen.

While in a standing posture, rest the arms along the sides of the body. Move the body weight to the front third of the feet. While rotating the forearms outward and gently opening the chest, turn the head to the left looking slightly upward. Relax the hips keeping them as still as possible.

Inhale slowly and gently through rounded lips filling the mouth with air. Close the mouth and gather saliva. Exhale as the body returns to center, letting the arms relax and body weight move back to the heels. Swallow the saliva and air together. Follow the saliva and air with your Mind's eye to the center of the abdomen. Rest the Mind in the abdomen for 3 to 6 breaths. Repeat left and right 6 to 9 times.

6. Bending Forward to Open the Spine and Activate the Belt Vessel

This exercise helps open the Yin and Yang Meridians of the legs and circulates Qi in the extraordinary meridian called the Belt Vessel.

From the standing position, curl the spine forward starting with the neck one vertebrae at a time. Once in full spinal flexion, let the upper body hang down towards the earth for a moment - shoulders hang, arms hang, head hangs.

Inhale and, with the palms, gather Qi from the earth. Slowly curl back into an upright position moving the palms up the inside of the feet and legs to the center line of the body, up over the head and outward into an embracing the Universe posture.

As you straighten the body, exhale letting the arms drop down to the front, so the palms come to rest two fist widths away from the Lower Dantian. Extend Qi from the center of the palms and fingers into the Lower Dantian via the Sea of Qi Point located about three finger widths below the navel.

Inhale pointing the fingers towards the Sea of Qi Point, located just below the navel. As you exhale move the fingers around the body following the Belt Vessel trajectory to the Ming Men point at the center of the lower back. Palms and fingers always face the body. Extend Qi from the center of the palms and fingers into the Lower Dantian via the Ming Men.

As you exhale, curl the upper body down towards the earth, sliding the palms down the back of the legs to the heels. Hang down for a moment. As you inhale, gather Qi from the earth with the palms and rise once again to the upright position, palms following the Yin Meridians on the inside of the legs. Repeat 9 to 12 times.

7. Chakra Balancing

Inhale opening the chest. Gather Qi with the palms and bring the Qi towards the front of the body "breaststroke fashion". Exhale, arching the back and extending Qi to the major energy centers or Chakras one at a time.

At each point, visualize sending Qi through body to the corresponding Chakras centers at back of the body, arching and opening the spine for each point in the following sequence.

- Reproductive Organs area to tip of the Coccyx or GV 1
- Just below the navel to the Ming Men or GV 4
- Solar Plexus region to the Center of the Spine or GV 6
- Mid Chest Point to the Spirit Pathway or GV 11
- Base of throat to the Great Vertebrae located at the lower boarder of C7 or GV 14
- Mouth to the occipital protuberance at the Palace of Wind or GV 16
- Mid eyebrow point to the Jade Pillow or BL 9

Arch the back slightly and open the palms up and out to the sky, embracing the Universe, gathering Heaven's energy. Rise up on the toes. Feel the energy. Smile to the energy.

Straighten the back while coming back down onto the heels. Beam the energy with the palms down into the Crown Point. Lower the palms down the front of the body, guiding the Universal energy down the Ren Channel to the Lower Dan Tian.

When the hands pass in front of the forehead they adopt a lotus palm posture, moving down to the front of the Heart. Pivot the lotus palm while moving down to the abdomen so the hands come to rest in the form of a small triangle with the opening between the palms placed over the Lower Dan Tian. Put the Mind in the center of the abdomen. Repeat 3 to 6 times.

8. Opening the 12 Regular Meridians followed by the Three Centers Merge Meditation

The palms are over the Lower Dantian, thumbs and index finger touching, forming a triangle, thumbs resting on the navel. Move the body weight to the right leg, bending the knee slightly. Rotate the hips to the left 45 degrees. The supporting leg is full. The other leg is empty.

Let the empty leg step forward onto the heel. Move the body weight forward letting the front foot drop to the floor as it turns slightly inward. At the same time bring the hands to the front of the body in a prayer position.

Then open the palms to the Universe straightening the back leg, turning the hips to the front, and letting the back heel adjust accordingly.

Raise the back heel. Open the chest and the eyes wide. Smile with the Universe. Step back to the original position crossing the forearms with the palms facing the earth. Bend the knees with the forearms resting over the thighs in a half-sitting posture.

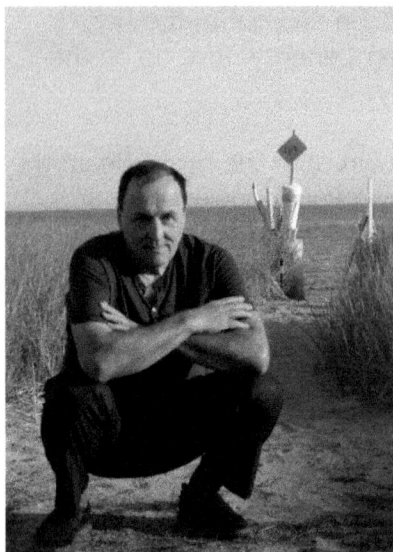

When in the sitting position, the heels stay in contact with the earth. If the heels start to lift before you reach the sitting position, stop and rest in a more upright position. When bending, the knees do not extend beyond the toes. Also, do not flex the back too far forward. The movement is like sitting on a chair. Drop the hips down, maintaining proper alignment of the shoulders, hips and center of feet. Relax while you practice Reverse Belly Breathing gently moving the energy up the back on inhalation and down the front on exhalation.

After a few moments, straighten the legs pushing the feet into the earth. As you stand, open the Crown Point towards the sky, and bring the palms back to the Lower Dantian thumbs and index fingers touching forming a triangle.

At this point practice **Three Centers Merge Meditation.** Let the awareness of the center of the brain where the pineal gland is located drop down to the center of the Lower Dantian. Let the center of the palms or Palace of Toil reach inward to the center of the Lower Dantian. Let the Bubbling Spring point on the soles of the feet reach upwards into the center of the Lower Dantian.

Let all three centers merge into the center of the Lower Dantian. Rest the Mind in the Lower Dantian for a few minutes before repeating the Opening the 12 Meridians Exercise on the opposite side. Repeat on both sides 6 to 9 times.

9. Rotating Trunk with Hands Tapping to Open the Hip Gate

Unresolved tension in the lower back area often impedes the free flow of Qi and Blood between the lower limbs and the upper body leading to stiffness and pain in the lumbar region. Sitting for long periods of time worsens this type of problem.

84

Arms hanging to the sides of the body, with a straight back, rotate the trunk from side to side. Let the arms move freely tapping the inguinal ligament at the front of the hips with one hand and the iliosacral joint on the lower back with the other hand.

Repeat 12 to 24 times. For the first repetitions keep the hips still. Then you can rotate both the trunk and hips to the side while tapping the hip gates.

10. Releasing the Lumbar Region

The Lumbar Eyes are located in visible hollows one hand width on either side of the lumbar spine, below the iliac crest. These points help strengthen the Kidneys and benefit the lumbar region. To activate these points, place the palms on the hips, thumbs facing the lumbar spine. Massage the Lumbar Eyes with the thumbs in a circular motion moving in towards the spine, down and back out. Repeat 9 to 18 times.

Move the hips forward extending the back at the hips and pressing the thumbs into the area being massaged. Bring the elbows closer together to help direct firm thumb pressure to the appropriate spot.

Gently place the tip of the tongue on the lower teeth. Smile from the Heart letting the mouth open slightly. Inhale through the mouth with a low hissing sound **Si..i..i..** Exhale through the mouth pronouncing the sound **Fu..u..u..** Feel the beating of the Heart in the lips as you exhale.

The **Fuu** sound blowing over the lips vibrates at the same rhythm as the Heart. This is very relaxing as it synchronizes the rhythm of the breath with the beating of the Heart. As always, let the chest drop during exhalation. The out breath is longer than the in breath. Breathe 3 to 6 times.

Bend the knees slightly moving the elbows towards the front to help open the hips and lower back. Let the chin drop down slightly towards the chest. Breathe 6 to 9 times with the healing sounds as before. Then lift the body to the upright position. At this point you may feel a rush of energy in the legs. Both exercises can be repeated up to 3 times.

This exercise helps release tension in the lower back and increases the flow of Qi below the knees by opening the Middle of the Crook or Bladder 40 point. This point is located at the back of the knee, at the center of the knee crease. Its activation benefits the lumbar region, legs and knees.

11. Lighting the Fire in the Lower Dantian with Reverse Belly Breathing

In Daoism the body is considered Yin and the eyes Yang. Look into the Lower Dantian to start the fire and heat up Yin. It takes two to three months for a regular person to feel heat in the Lower Dantian.

Do not think too much. Stay in the center of the Lower Dantian for a few minutes but do not stare. Use the Mind's eye to plant the Qi seed and let it grow without effort.

The following exercise helps further energize the Lower Dantian. It involves reverse breathing and the gentle lifting of the anus and perineum. It is good for increasing sexual energy, for premature ejaculation, and for preventing prolapsed of the anus, uterus and Stomach. It is good for the excretory system and helps prevent hemorrhoids, colon cancer and localized infections. It can be combined with the practice of the Microcosmic Orbit Meditation.

Feet together, heels touching, move 70% of the body's weight to the front third of the feet. Bring the palms to navel. Women right hand first, men left hand first. The hands can also rest in any position.

Inhale contracting the abdomen and gently lifting the anus. Exhale and relax, bringing the Mind to the Lower Dantian. Repeat 10 to 50 times.

On inhalation, visualize the energy moving in a circular fashion, like the turning of a wheel, from the navel to the Hui Yin to the Ming Men and back to the navel where you exhale and relax.

Movement creates energy. If a space does not move it becomes stagnant and problems can occur. Reverse Belly Breathing creates a smaller space in the abdomen. It massages the organs and creates more energy.

It is a powerful exercise so proceed with caution starting with only 10 repetitions and increasing repetitions slowly over time to up to 50 per session.

12. Shaking Method with Cleansing Breath

Everyone has tired or stagnant energy. The shaking method helps to dislodge toxic Qi and separate the vibrant from the stagnant Qi. The body warms up if the exercise is done properly.

Drop the hands down the sides of body. Bounce lightly, bending and extending the knees shaking the whole body. Make sure every area of the body shakes. Practice the shaking method for 5 minutes.

While shaking, relax each part of the body: Head; Shoulders; Neck, Arms, Forearms, and Hands, Chest; Abdomen; Hips; Groin, and Legs.

The **Circular Three Level Shaking Method** can eventually be incorporated into the routine. Stop shaking the whole body and focus on rotating the hips back and forth, then the rib cage ending with the neck and head. Repeat 3 times. Do not attempt this method if you suffer from any type of neck weakness. After a few shakes return to the original full-body shaking method.

At the end of the method, visualize breathing pure universal energy in through the Crown of the head into the abdomen. Then breathe stagnant Qi out the legs and feet deep into the earth. Repeat 6 to 9 times.

Bring the palms to the lower abdomen and the Mind to the center of Lower Dantian. Rest the Mind there for a moment. This brings Qi to the lower Dantian.

13. Three Line Method to Relax the Body

In this method, we inhale through the Bai Hui or Crown Point down the center core of the body or Tai Chi Pole and exhale out down the outside of the body to the feet.

This method is very relaxing. It harmonizes the Wei Qi or protective bio-energy field which radiates out from the exterior of the body.

Stand in the Wu Ji or Standing-on-Posts posture with the arms hanging down the sides of the body. Inhale universal energy into the Bai Hui or Crown Point of the head into the center of the body down to the Lower Dantian. Exhale Qi out the center core via the Bai Hui down the front of the body along the Conception Vessel and legs to the toes. Repeat 3 to 6 times.

Inhale universal energy into the Bai Hui or Crown Point of the head into the center of the body down to the Lower Dantian. Exhale Qi out the Bai Hui down the sides of body to the feet. Repeat 3 to 6 times.

Inhale universal energy into the Bai Hui or Crown Point of the head into the center of the body down to the Lower Dantian. Exhale Qi out the Bai Hui down the back of the body along the Governor Vessel, and down the back of the legs to the heels. Repeat 3 to 6 times.

Inhale universal energy into the Bai Hui or Crown Point of the head into the center of the body down to the Lower Dantian. Exhale Qi out the Bai Hui down the front, sides and back of body to the feet. Repeat 3 to 6 times.

14. Standing on Posts with Whole Body Breathing

Stand with the feet shoulder width apart. Imagine the palms are holding a balloon or Qi ball in front of the lower abdomen. The hands are located about two fist widths away from the abdomen, at the same level as the Sea of Qi Point located just below the navel.

Practice Pores or Whole-Body Breathing. Breathe in universal energy through the pores of the skin into the center of the abdomen and exhale out far into the Universe. Practice for 10 to 20 minutes. Normally, 30 breaths equal approximately 5 minutes of practice.

15. Tai Chi Walk

Holding a Qi ball in front of the lower abdomen, shift the body weight to one leg. Turn the hips towards the opposite corner and step out with the front leg placing the heel on the floor. Then as you shift the weight of the body forward, drop the front foot onto the floor, turning the toes in slightly.

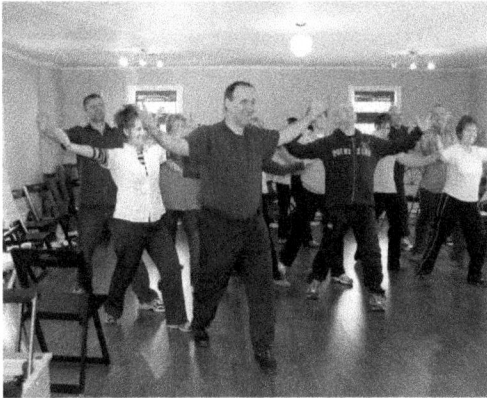

As you inhale, rotate the hips to the front, opening the arms and eyes wide to embrace the Universe. Exhale while you bring the palms back to center, stepping forward with the back leg onto the ball of the foot, which is placed next the center of the supporting foot, hip width apart. Both knees are slightly bent to avoid moving the body up and down while you step.

Turn the hips to the opposite corner and step out to the heel, repeating the same movement but on the opposite side. Stay relaxed and attentive as you walk for about 5 minutes. Experience the opening and closing of the torso as you inhale and exhale.

16. Natural Walking Qi Gong with Whole Body Breathing

It is better to practice Natural Walking Qi Gong in a clean natural environment. When walking open the Ming Men by curling the tail bone under as if sitting on a chair.

Imagine that the crown of the head is suspended from above. Relax the body. Move from heel to ball of foot pulling the body forward with the front foot once it lays flat on the floor or ground. The

89

opposite leg and arm move at the same time. The arms swing naturally back and forth along the sides of the body. Once the walk becomes natural, add Whole Body Breathing to the exercise. The Natural Walk can be done every day as you go about your regular activities.

17. Fixed Step Qi Gong

Stand feet shoulder width apart. Bend the knees as if you were sitting on a chair and scoop up Qi from the front of the body with the palms facing upward. Bring the Qi to the chest area. When the hands reach the mid chest area, rotate the forearms outward so the backs of the hands are facing each other.

Extend the hands forward to the front of the body and then in a continuous movement out to a T-Stance. Bring the hands down to the sides of the body and start again. Repeat 6 to 9 times.

18. Self Massage

 The form ends with a massage of the abdomen, face and head. The abdominal massage helps consolidate the Qi in the lower abdomen and descend rebellious Qi helping resolve digestive issues, calming the Liver and the Spleen.

The facial massage beautifies the skin and releases tension in the neck and head area. The head massage strengthens the ears and Kidneys and helps open the Palace of Wind energy gate located at the back of the head just below the occipital protuberance.

- Bring the palms to the navel. Men place right hand over left, women left hand over right.
- Massage the abdomen in a circular fashion 9 times in each direction. Increase the size of the rotations as you turn the palms towards the left. During this movement, the palms remain between the pubic bone and the sternum. Once you change directions, reduce the size of the rotations ending at the starting point over the navel.
- Raise the hands to the center of the chest and massage the centerline of the body with the heels of the hands down to the pubic bone. Repeat 9 to 18 times.

- Separate the palms and place them on the floating ribs. Massage down to the pubic bone. Repeat 9 to 18 times.
- Bring the hands to the front of the body, palms together. Rub the palms together vigorously and place them over the front of the face, fingers pointing towards the sky.
- Massage the face by moving hands to the back of the head so the thumb and index fingers touch. Repeat 6 to 9 times.
- Rake the centerline of the head with the tips of the fingers 3 to 6 times.
- With the ears placed between the middle and index fingers, massage the sides of the ears by moving the hands up and down 50 to 100 times.
- Massage the ears by pressing the thumbs against the ears three times.
- With the thumb and sides of the index fingers, pull the ears out and then down.
- Pop the ears 3 times by placing the middle fingers in the ear opening, twisting the fingers twice in the same direction, and releasing.
- Drum the Qi by placing the cupped palms over the ears with the fingers lying on the back of the head. Drum 3 sets of 9 for each of the three following methods – alternating fingers, all fingers together, snapping middle finger over ring finger.
- Drop the palms to throat level, finger pads resting below the ears on the jaw line. In a twisting motion gently massage the front of the throat with the base of the palms with alternating hands. Repeat 9 times. Repeat the same movement but with both hands 9 times.

19. Relaxation with Soong

Move Qi down the front of the body with the palms and release stagnant Qi deep into the earth. Gather Qi with the palms and place them over the abdomen, thumbs overlapping slightly at the navel, men right hand over left, and women left hand over right.

Use the Mind to expand the body outward as big as the Universe. Inhale observing universal Qi enter the body. Exhale with the sound SOONG vibrating the nose and whole body from head to toes. Repeat 3 to 6 times.

Medical Qi Gong

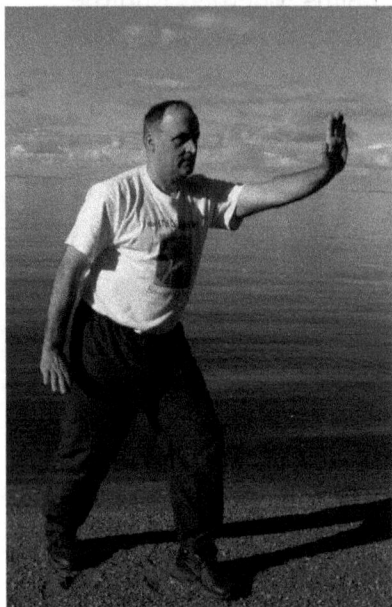

Specialized Qi Gong forms are available to help prevent or resolve many disorders such as myopia, frequent urination, lower back pain, anxiety, digestive issues, respiratory distress, high blood pressure, varicose veins and cancer to name but a few.

To help you understand how these exercises work, I have included in this presentation exercise routines for:
- **Digestive Issues**
- **High and Low Blood Pressure**
- **Respiratory Disorders**
- **Anxiety**

Qi Gong for Digestive Issues

An increasing number of people suffer from digestive and excretory problems. This style of Qi Gong is especially helpful in invigorating and regulating digestion.

Studies have shown that the up-and-down movements of the diaphragm muscles are much larger with Qi Gong practitioners than in those who do not practice Qi Gong. The unique breathing methods used by Qi Gong effectively expand the amplitude of diaphragm movements, which in turn strengthen the massaging function on the Intestines and Stomach.

The upper portion of the Stomach of a Qi Gong practitioner was also found to be six times higher than that of a non-practitioner. These Qi Gong related changes prevent diseases of the gastrointestinal tract as well as premature aging.

Qi Gong exercises also help regulate peristalsis and influence the secretion of the digestive glands. Unlike general Qi Gong styles, you can practice Qi Gong for digestive issues right after eating, even after a big meal, to help ease discomfort in the Stomach.

This style helps relieve problems in the abdominal area, such as diabetes, irritable bowel syndrome, constipation, diarrhea, abdominal pains, bloating, gas, belching, stomach problems and more.

1. Open with the Universe Meditation

Sitting on the front third of a chair, open the legs to shoulder width, parallel to each other and perpendicular to the floor. Rest the back of the wrists on the thighs above the knees, palms facing up. Palms face down if you suffer from High Blood Pressure.

Move the chin slightly inward towards the Adams apple, with the crown of head suspended from above. Place the tongue gently on the upper palate, behind the upper front teeth. The eyes are open, or half closed, the anus gently closed. Relax the body front and back, head to toes, one section at a time.

Using the Mind expand the part of the body you are focusing on as big as the Universe. Inhale letting universal energy enter the body. Then exhale and relax.

Section 1: Eyebrows; Sides of Head; Shoulders; Elbows; Wrists; Fingers; Middle Finger

Section 2: Face; Throat; Chest; Abdomen; Reproductive Organs; Pelvic Floor; Hips; Knees; Ankles; Toes; Big Toe

Section 3: Back of Head; Upper Back; Lower Back; Tail Bone; Back of Knees; Heels; Soles of Feet (Bubbling Spring)

To end the sequence, use the Mind to expand the whole body outward on inhalation as big as the Universe. Visualize expanding every cell outward as big at the Universe, then every molecule, photons and particles. Repeat each section 9 times.

Bring the palms to the Lower Dantian, thus bringing Qi to the abdomen. Rest your Mind in the abdomen for a few minutes. Meditation is important as it opens your natural healing abilities. The Universe is within you. You are the Universe. Be happy and relax with the Universe.

2. Relaxed Belly Breathing with Lifting of Anus

Inhale 70% of respiratory capacity while expanding the abdomen outward and gently lifting the anus. Then exhale 100% of capacity while relaxing the abdomen and anus.

As you inhale visualize energy moving up the center of the body from the pelvic floor to the Crown Point located on the top of the head. Relax as you exhale. To facilitate practice, you may inhale to the count of seven and exhale to the count of ten. Repeat 10 to 50 times.

3. Swallow Saliva or the Pill of Immortality

Place the palms over the lower Dantian, men left hand first, women right hand first. The mouth is closed, with the tip of the tongue placed on the top of the palate. Practice natural breathing for a few moments.

- Click the teeth together gently on the left side of the mouth then on the right side 12 times
- Click all the teeth together gently 12 times
- Turn the tongue in a left circle inside of the teeth area 9 times
- Turn the tongue in a right circle outside of the teeth area 9 times
- Use the tongue to touch roof of the mouth 3 times, the bottom 3 times, and the center between the front teeth 3 times.
- Inhale gathering the saliva accumulated in the mouth.
- Exhale and swallow the saliva following it with the Mind's eye down to the Lower Dantian. Repeat swallowing the saliva 3 times.

4. Stimulate Acupoints

According to Chinese Medicine, the following acupoints are very effective in stimulating Qi along the meridians involved in digestive issues. Even if you press the wrong points, they will not produce negative side effects. Skip doing the acupoints if you feel uncomfortable with them.

- Joining Valley or Large Intestine 4 (LI 4) located on the back of the hand at the midpoint of the second metacarpal bone along the radial border. Regulates upward and downward movement of Qi. Improves intestinal function, constipation and abdominal pain.

- Inner Pass or Pericardium 5 (PE 5) located on the inner forearm approximately three thumb widths above the wrist crease. Relieves Stomach aches, indigestion and vomiting.

- Middle Cavity or Ren 12 located halfway between the breastbone and belly button, on the midline of the body. Relieves heartburn, indigestion and abdominal pain.

- Central Courtyard or Ren 16 located at the level of the sternocostal angle on the midline of the sternum. Lowers rebellious Stomach Qi and relieves belching, food stagnation and nausea.

- Spirit Storehouse or Kidney 25 (Kid 25) located between the sternum and mamillary line in the second intercostal space. Lowers rebellious Lung and Stomach Qi. Treats belching. Opens the chest.

- Heaven's Pivot or Stomach 25 (ST 25) located about two thumb widths lateral to the belly button. These points help relieve constipation, abdominal pain and digestive disorders.

- Leg Three Miles or Stomach 36 (ST 36) located on the lateral side of the legs approximately one palm width below the knee. Helps relieve nausea, gas and bloating.

- Points on the Liver, Stomach and Gall Bladder meridians located on the top of feet help relieve nausea, vomiting and abdominal pain.

On the LI 4, PE 5 and Kid 25, using the thumb pad rotate in both directions 9 times or more while applying pressure. Then press inward with the thumb while inhaling, and release pressure on exhalation. Keep the joints of the thumb rounded to avoid injury and improve energy flow. When pressing on the point, visualize energy going to the organ that belongs to the meridian being activated. Repeat 9 times or more.

On Ren 12, Ren 16 and ST 25 use the pads of the fingers of one hand to massage the area in both directions 9 times or more while applying light pressure. The second hand can overlap the first to help apply even pressure. Then press inward with the finger pads while inhaling, and release pressure on exhalation. Repeat 9 to 12 times.

On the ST 36 points and top of the feet you can use the heel of the opposite leg to friction the areas for a few minutes.

5. Harmonize Liver and Triple Warmer with Healing Sounds

Place the left palm on the navel and the right palm over the Liver. On inhalation visualize the Liver and its healthy pearl green color. On exhalation pronounce the Liver healing sound **"Shu...e...e"**. Repeat 9 or more times.

Place the right palm over the Heart. On inhalation visualize the Triple Warmer, which encompasses the digestive and excretory systems, and its healthy orange red color. On exhalation pronounce the Triple Warmer healing sound **"She...e...e..."**. Repeat 9 more times. (For more information refer to the section on Healing Sounds)

6. Harmonize the Liver to Appease the Spleen with Eye Qi Gong

The eyes are the opening of the Liver to the exterior world. Therefore, by exercising the eyes, we help bring the Liver system back into balance. The Liver is the great harmonizer of emotions. Calming the Liver helps relieve stress, frontal headaches and anxiety.

Disharmony of the Liver Organ System often leads to digestive issues as an unhappy Liver may encroach on the Stomach and Spleen negatively affecting their normal functions of transforming and transporting food.

The extraocular muscles of the eyes can be exercised like any other muscle in the body. The eyes can be moved from side to side, up and down and in a circular motion. With practice they can also be moved back and forth in the eye socket.

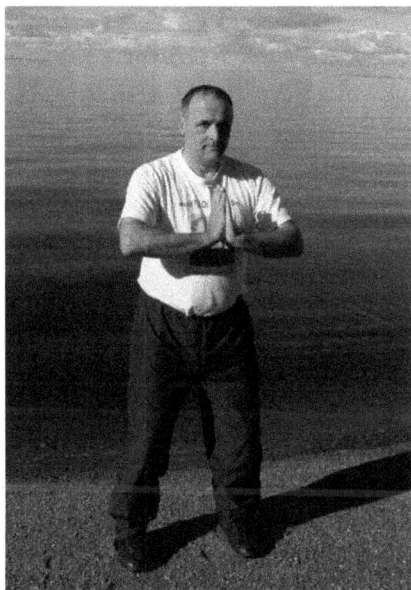

Bring the palms together with the fingers pointing upwards, thumbs facing the Chest Center, one-fist width away from the body, with forearms parallel to the earth. Smile from the Heart.

First Part - Eye Exercises

- **Eyes closed:** As you inhale, move the eyeballs forward looking far out to the horizon. As you exhale, move the eyeballs back into the eye socket looking far back to the horizon. Repeat 28 times.

- **Eyes open:** As you inhale move the eyeballs forward looking far out to the horizon. As you exhale, close the eyelids, and move the eyeballs back into the eye socket looking far back to the horizon. Repeat 28 times.

During these first two exercises, imagine the horizon forming an unbroken circle around the head.

- **Eyes closed:** Inhale rolling the eyes in a "U" from the left corner of the eyes to the bottom, across the bottom and up to the right corner. Exhale rolling the eyes in the opposite direction. Repeat 28 times.

- Eyes open: Keep the eyes open without blinking for 6 breaths. For an additional 6 breaths open the eyes wide on each inhalation and on exhalation relax the eyes keeping them open throughout the whole exercise without blinking.

- Eyes closed: Rub the palms together until they feel warm and place them over the forehead and the eyes. Practice relaxed belly breathing for a few moments.

Second Part - Stretching Qi

With the palms facing each other one fist width away from the mid-chest area, inhale opening the hands to the width of the face. Then on exhalation close the hands to the width of the nose. Repeat 9 to 18 times.

Inhale opening the hands to the width of the shoulders. Close the hands to the width of the head. Repeat 9 to 18 times.

Third Part - Self Massage

With the middle, ring and little fingers gently flexed, activate the following pressure points with the pads of the index fingers. Place the finger pads on the points. Inhale applying light pressure while sending Qi into the point. Exhale and relax. Repeat 6 to 12 times.

1. Inner corner of the eyes at BL 1 or Bright Eyes
2. Center of the eyebrows at Yu Yao or Fish Waist
3. At the exterior of eyes at GB 1 or Pupil Crevice
4. Below the cheek bones at ST 2 or Four Whites

With the thumbs, massage two pressure points at the back of the head located at GB 12 just below the ears on the Mastoid Process, and at BL 10 just below the occipital protuberance.

With the thumb pads on the points, inhale applying light pressure while sending Qi into the point. Exhale and relax. Repeat 6 to 12 times.

While holding the forehead with one palm, massage the Big Vertebrae located at T1 in a circular motion with the pads of the fingers. Then pinch the back of the neck between the thumb and fingers from the Big Vertebrae to the occipital protuberance. Switch hands and repeat the exercise.

7. Building Qi Between the Palms

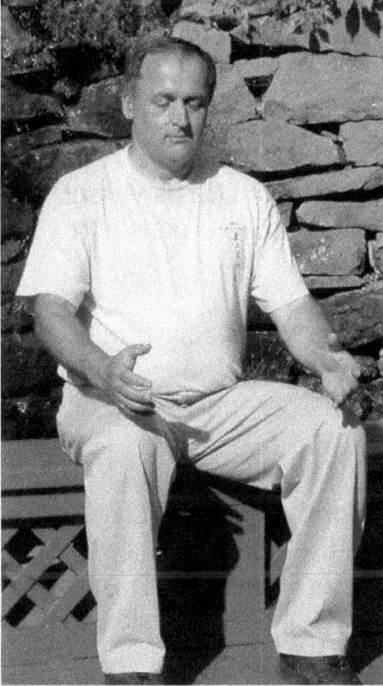

The following exercises build strong Qi between the palms improving the effectiveness of the Raising the Palms to Regulate or Smooth the Qi style.

Grinding Qi: The palms face each other fist-width apart, in front of the lower abdomen. Move the hands in a circular motion grinding the Qi. Focus the Mind on the center of the palms. Move as fast as you can comfortably 30 to 50 times. Breathe naturally.

Pulling Qi: The palms face each other about the width of the head in front of the lower abdomen. Focus the Mind on the center of the palms. As you inhale (70% of respiratory capacity), open the palms to about the width of the shoulders. As you exhale (100% of respiratory capacity), return the palms to the original position. Repeat 9 to 12 times.

8. Raising the Palms to Regulate or Smooth the Qi

This exercise helps clear out dense Qi and re-establish energy flow and balance. It smooths the Qi in the Stomach, Liver and Spleen meridians that run along the front of the chest and abdomen improving the digestive function. Stand with palms facing the lower abdomen fingers pointing towards each other. Hands are about two fists-width away from the body.

Inhale, turning the left forearm slightly upward while lifting it to shoulder height. Exhale and turn the left palm slightly downward, returning it to navel height. Repeat 9 times.

Without moving the left hand, repeat the same movement with the right hand 9 times. Then on inhalation, lift both palms to shoulder height. Exhale, lowering the palms to navel height. Repeat 9 times. Focus the Mind on regulating or smoothing the Qi on the front of the body.

9. Turning the Water Wheel

This exercise moves Qi up the center core of the body where resides the Chung or Penetrating Vessel and the Bao Mai or Uterus Vessel. These two energy pathways connect the reproductive organs and Kidneys with the Heart.

In a person suffering from rebellious Qi of the digestive system the increased upward pressure in the Stomach moves up the center core of the body via these channels affecting the proper functioning of the Heart.

With the palms facing each other the width of the hips apart, move the hands down and out, up and back down the front of the body in a circular movement like the turning of a water wheel. Inhale as the palms move down, out and up the shoulder height and exhale as the palms move down the front of the body.

On inhalation expand the abdomen and raise the anus gently imagining the Qi moving up the center core of the body to the crown point. On exhalation relax and let go of tension. Repeat 9 to 12 times.

10. Open the Spleen Meridian

This is one example of a stretching exercise that opens the meridian of an organ system which plays an important role in the digestive function. This exercise helps open the Spleen Meridian and balance its energy thus improving digestion and energy generated from acquired Qi.

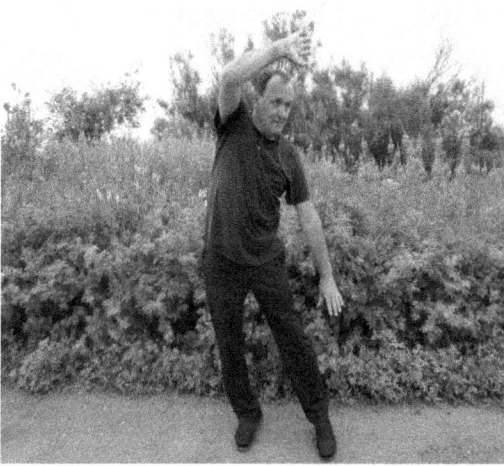

Inhale, moving the hands to the front of the body as if holding a ball encompassing the area in front of the body from the navel to the bottom end of the sternum. The left hand is on the bottom, the right hand on the top, with the palms facing each other. Turn the energy ball around for a few moments to help generate more Qi.

Move 70 percent of the body weight to the right leg. Raise the left heel off the ground moving the hips laterally towards the supporting leg. Exhale, extending the left palm down the side of the left leg, and the right palm upwards towards the sky. The body is in the shape of a bow.

Inhale, lowering the heel, returning the extended leg back to its original position, arms to a "T" stance and then into the holding-the-energy-ball posture but with the right palm on the bottom and the left on top. Repeat the same movement on the opposite site. Repeat the sequence again on both sides 6 to 9 times.

11. Open the Triple Warmer

The Triple Warmer or San Jiao is not an organ system but encompasses three body cavities which contain all the organs of the body. The cavities correspond to the areas located at the level of the hips, floating ribs and shoulders. According to the classic Chinese Medical text "Simple Questions" the Triple Warmer is the official in charge of irrigation and it controls the water passages affecting both the distribution of Qi and body fluids.

To open the Triple Warmer, stand feet shoulder width apart, with the arms resting along the sides of the body. Bend the knees slightly while breathing into the **hip area**. At the same time, lift the arms from the sides of the body the distance of approximately two fist widths. Exhale straightening the knees while moving the palms back to their original position. Repeat 6 to 9 times.

While flexing the knees, breathe into the **floating ribs**. At the same time, let the palms move away from the sides of the body the distance of approximately four fist widths. Exhale straightening the knees slightly while lowering the palms to their original position. Repeat 6 to 9 times.

Finally, bend the knees while breathing into the **shoulder area**. At the same time, raise the arms up the sides of the body approximately six fist widths or shoulder height. Exhale straightening the knees slightly while lowering the palms to their original position. Repeat 6 to 9 times.

12. Meditation on Spleen Yin organ via the Back Shu and Front Mu AcuPoints

The Spleen front Mu points are located at the Liver 13 acupoints which are at elbow height – on the lateral side of the abdomen, below the free end of the eleventh floating rib. The Spleen back Shu points are located along the spine at the level of Thoracic Vertebrae 11 a thumb width and a half outward from the spinal column at Bladder 20 which is slightly higher than Liver 13.

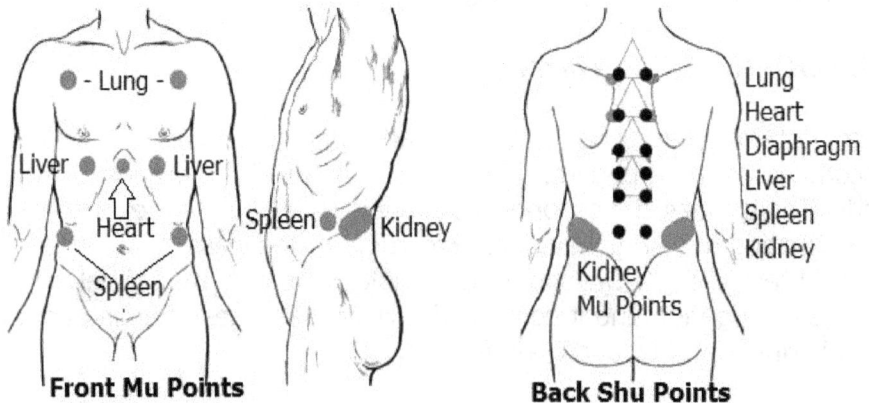

Front Mu Points   **Back Shu Points**

When meditating on Yin organs such as the Spleen first visualize and inhale into the Spleen Yang Back Shu points and exhale out far into the distance. Repeat 12 times.

102

Then visualize and inhale into the Spleen Front Mu points and exhale out far into the distance. Repeat 12 times.

Then visualize and inhale into both the Spleen Shu and Mu Points simultaneously, and exhale far out into the distance. Repeat 12 times.

13. Closing with Self Massage and SOONG

Hands resting on the navel - ladies right hand under, left over, men left hand under, right over.

- With natural breathing turn the hands in spiral movements 9 times in both directions.
- Move hands left to right on the abdomen.
- Move hands from the solar plexus to the pubic bone.
- Move hands from the floating ribs to the pubic bone.
- Move hands in a figure EIGHT "8"
- Rub palms vigorously
- Place hands on the face with the fingers pointing to the sky and wipe the hands back over the face to the sides of the head six times
- Bend the fingers and brush back vigorously over the eyebrows to the back of the head six times
- Drop the palms down to the navel collecting Qi
- Relax and rest the Mind in the lower abdomen for a few moments
- Imagine the whole body is as big as the Universe. Inhale letting the universal energy enter the body. Exhale pronouncing the healing sound SOONG vibrating the nose and body from head to toes 3 to 6 times

Qi Gong for Regulating Blood Pressure

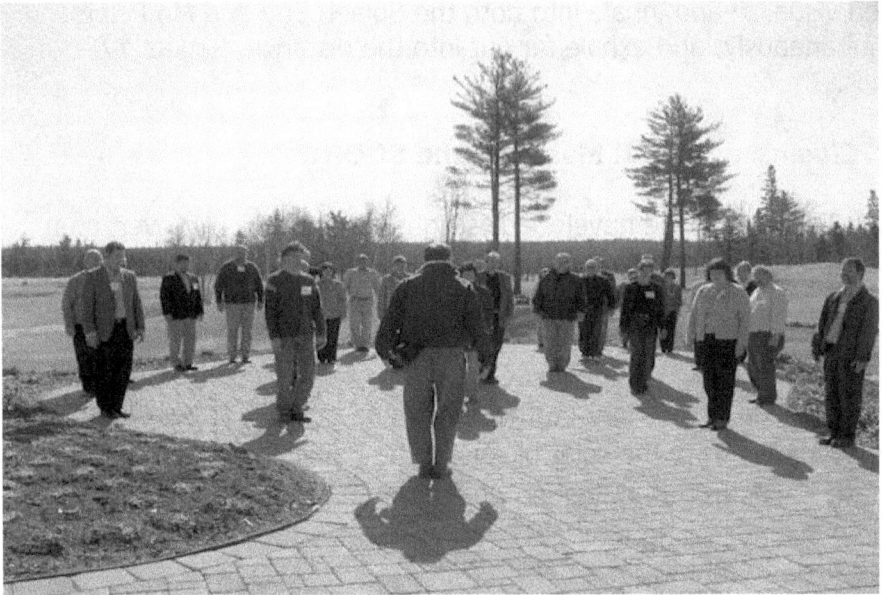

In China, the application of Qi Gong therapy in the prevention and treatment of hypertension has a history of more than 40 years. The Shanghai Institute of Hypertension treated 516 patients of hypertension with Qigong for one year with a total efficiency of 86.2%. (Source: Geneva Foundation for Medical Education and Research - www.gfmer.ch)

The Beijing Traditional Chinese Medicine Hospital reported that they treated 136 cases of hypertension with "Standing Qi Gong". An impressive 91.9% of the cases responded to the treatment. It is generally considered that Qi Gong lowers high blood pressure mainly by regulating the whole body, especially by regulating the functions of the central nervous system.

When practiced every day this style of Qi Gong regulates high and low blood pressure. The exercises can be done sitting or standing. General Qi Gong practice also helps regulate blood pressure.

When practicing Qi Gong for regulation of blood pressure always consult with your Medical Doctor concerning intake of medications related to this condition.

1. Relaxation with SOONG

For High Blood Pressure, first adopt a standing posture with the following indications:

- Feet shoulder width apart with 70% of body weight on the heels
- Knees straight but soft
- Abdomen pressed gently against the lower back
- Chin gently moving in and upward
- Arms hang down the sides of the body with palms of hands open and facing the body about one fist-width away
- Anus is closed gently and the tip of the tongue is placed on the upper palate behind the front teeth
- Eyes are fully open or half closed
- Practice with soft eyes looking towards the horizon

Use the Mind to open different parts of the body as big as the Universe. Start with the head, followed by the neck, shoulders, chest, abdomen, upper back, lower back, arms/hands and fingers, hips and groin area, and finally the legs/feet and toes.

On inhalation let universal Qi enter the part of the body you are focusing on. On exhalation, pronounce the healing sound SOONG letting the Qi condense in that area of the body. When pronouncing the word SOONG, let the nose vibrate with the healing sound as well as the part of the body you are focusing on.

Then repeat the exercise but for the whole body from head to toes three times. Repeat the sequence if required.

For Low Blood Pressure, adopt a sitting position with the wrists resting on the thighs, palms facing up.

Relax each part of the body as indicted in the previous exercise making the sound SOONG when exhaling. Relax the head, neck, shoulders, chest, abdomen, upper back, lower back, arms/hands and fingers, hips and groin area, legs/feet and toes. Then relax whole body from head to toes 3 times. Repeat if required.

2. Relaxed Belly Breathing

Inhale through the nose, to the count of seven, expanding the lower part of the body, front, side and back. Exhale through the nose to the count of ten letting the chest drop. Repeat 10 to 30 times.

The breath is gentle, silent, slow, deep and unbroken. Let the inhalation rise on its own from the space between exhalation and inhalation. Thirty breaths equal about five minutes.

Patients with High Blood Pressure should relax in the standing posture for an additional 5 minutes. Practice natural breathing with the Mind resting in the feet to help the body's energy descend towards the earth.

3. Open and Close Arms to Collect Qi

Place the hands in front of the navel palms facing each other about the width of the nose. Feel the Qi between the palms. Open the arms to about shoulder width. As you inhale let the abdomen expand opening the arms. As you exhale let the abdomen contract closing the arms. Repeat 9 to 12 times.

4. Project Qi to Bai Hui (Crown of Head)

After feeling or pulling the Qi between the palms, bring the hands down to the sides of body. Gather more Qi by opening the hands outward 45 degrees. Raise the hands above the head over the Bai Hui or Crown Point.

Palms are facing the top of the head. Fingers are pointing towards each other but do not touch. Keep the wrists relaxed and straight. Inhale as you raise and exhale as you lower the hands using the

Mind to project Qi to the Bai Hui 6 to 9 times. Use no strength or effort.

To lower Blood Pressure:
- As you raise the hands, visualize normal blood pressure. As you lower the hands, visualize blood pressure lowering.

To raise Blood Pressure:
- As you raise the hands, visualize blood pressure rising. As you lower the hands, visualize normal blood pressure.

Bring the middle fingers to the Bai Hui, back of hands touching, palms facing outward. Rotate the fingers three times in each direction applying gentle pressure with the middle finger sending Qi to the area. When turning the fingers, depending on your condition, visualize blood pressure increasing or decreasing. Repeat 12 times.

5. Interlocking Fingers (Middle finger Heart Meridian)

After completing the previous movement, open the palms and bring the hands down to the navel. If you have been sitting, adopt a standing Posture. The legs are open shoulder width, feet parallel, knees slightly bent. Interlock fingers, with the middle fingers pointing

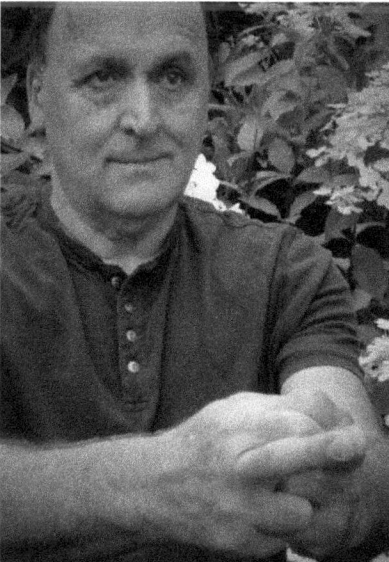

out, thumbs folded over each other and hidden inside the palms. Bring the palms together.

A. Point the end of the middle fingers to the Yin Tang (Center of Eyebrows) and rotate to the left while pronouncing the healing sound Xing (**Sing**) three times. Rotate the fingers to the right while pronouncing same healing sound three times.

B. Point the end of the middle fingers at the center of the chest and rotate to the left while pronouncing the healing sound Xien

107

(**Seanne**) three times. Rotate the fingers to the right pronouncing same healing sound three times.

C. Extend the arms outward to the front of the chest. Point the end of the fingers away from body and rotate with small movements to the left while pronouncing the healing sound **Shen** three times. Rotate fingers to the right while pronouncing the healing sound **Shen** three times. Repeat the A, B and C sequence 3 times in total.

This movement helps regulate the heart.

During the exercises always visualize either increasing or reducing Blood Pressure depending on what is required.

6. Cool Down for High Blood Pressure

Relax the arms and move them down to the sides of the body. Then raise the arms away from the sides of the body turning the palms up. Visualize holding cold ice as you raise the arms upward as people with High Blood Pressure are hot.

Carry the ice to the top of the head, palms facing the Bai Hui or Crown Point. Let the cool water pour over the body. Lower the hands down the front of the body while visualizing lowering High Blood Pressure. From the chin level, down to the navel visualize Normal Blood Pressure. Repeat 9 to 12 times.

7. Harmonize the Kidneys & the Heart

According to the Five Element Theory the Kidneys represent the Water element and the Heart represents the Fire element. The Kidney Water helps cool or regulate the Heart Fire and the Heart Fire helps heat up the Kidney Water.

Each organ system depends on the other to help maintain a state of balance. The following exercise helps regulate the connection between these two organ systems.

Place the left hand above the Heart with the palm facing the chest, about a fist width away from the body. Place the right hand above the Lower Dantian, about a fist width away from the body.

Breathe naturally for a few minutes, letting the Mind focus on the Heart Fire. Feel the heat radiating from the Heart to the palms. Then continue breathing for a few minutes letting the Mind focus on the Kidneys. Feel the coolness radiating from the Kidneys to the palms.

Then switch hand positions. For a few minutes focus on cooling the Heart Fire with the Kidney Water and then warming the Kidney Water with the Heart Fire. Repeat 3 to 6 times. Switch the hands again and focus on normalizing the Heart Fire and Kidney Water.

8. Closing

If standing, bring the feet together so the heels touch lightly.
- Collect Qi, open arms out and rest the palms just below the navel. Ladies: right hand under, left over. Men: left hand under, right over. Rest the Mind in the center of the abdomen.
- Turn the hands in a spiraling movement 9 times to the left and then to the right.
- Rub the hands vigorously 9 times.
- Put the hands over the face, breathe in, and on inhalation slide the hands over the face to the sides and back of the head 6 times.
- Bend the fingers, breathe in, and as you exhale brush back hard over the eyebrows to the back of the head with the fingers 6 times.
- Lower the palms and collect Qi to the navel
- Relax and SOONG head to toes 6 times.

Qi Gong for Respiratory Disorders

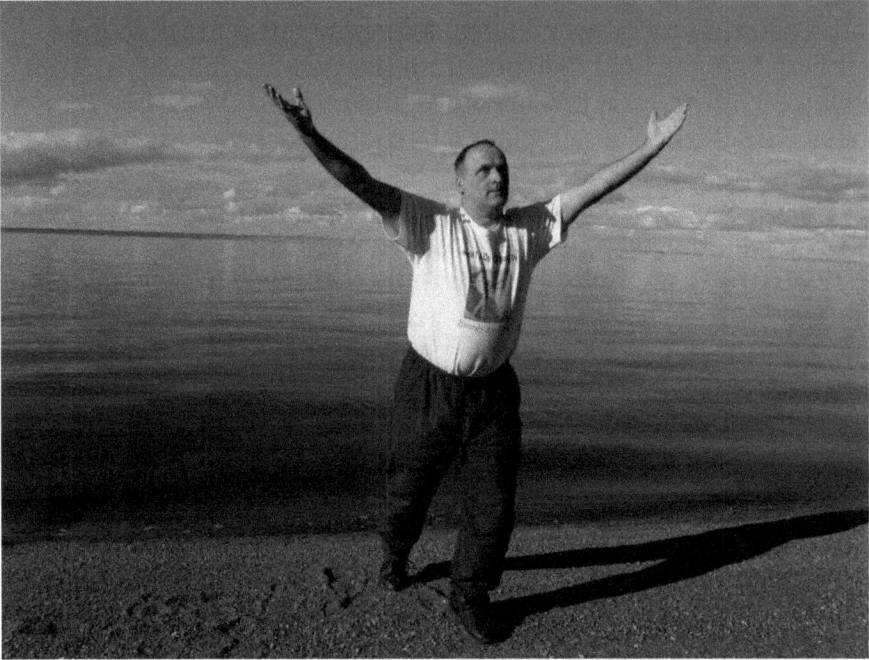

This form helps prevent respiratory disorders such as shortness of breath, asthma and frequent colds by eliminating stagnant Qi from the Lungs, and by strengthening the air passageways, Lungs and Heart.

1. Relax with SOONG

Sit on the edge of a chair feet shoulder width apart. Arms are rounded, palms facing up with the back of hands resting on the thighs above the knees. The head is level, chin slightly in and back straight.

Still the body and quiet the Mind. Relax the back, chest and waist. Gently place the tip of the tongue on the palate behind upper front teeth. Close the anal sphincter. Eyes are open or half closed.

Use the Mind to open different parts of the body as big as the Universe. Inhale letting universal Qi enter the body. On exhalation pronounce the healing sound SOONG. When pronouncing the word SOONG, let the nose vibrate with the healing sound as well as the part of the body you are focusing on.

SOONG the head, neck, shoulders, chest, abdomen, upper back, lower back, arms/hands and fingers, hips and groin area, legs/feet and toes. Then SOONG the whole body from head to toes 6 times. Repeat if necessary.

2. Relaxed Belly Breathing

Inhale and exhale through the nose. The breath is thin, even, silent, deep and long. Inhale expanding the abdomen outward in all directions, exhale letting the chest drop down towards the hips.

Do not force the inhalation. Inhale 70% of respiratory capacity, and exhale 100%. Be aware of the quiet space between exhalation and inhalation. Let the inhalation rise on its own from this quiet space. Practice 30 breaths or for 5 minutes.

3. Opening the Air Passageways with Dental Qi Gong

The ancients believed that saliva contains special antiseptic properties that kill germs in the digestive track helping prevent respiratory disease. Saliva was called the **The Pill of Immortality** as it also helps strengthen the Jing Qi or essential essence located in the Lower Dantian.

In a sitting or standing position:

- Click the front teeth together lightly 9 times
- Click the left row of the teeth lightly 9 times
- Click the right row of the teeth lightly 9 times
- Click all the teeth together lightly 9 times
- Turn the tongue to the left in a circular motion behind the teeth gathering saliva 9 times

- Turn the tongue to the right in a circular motion in front of the teeth gathering saliva 9 times
- Tap the tip of the tongue against the upper palate 3 times
- Tap the tip of the tongue against the lower front teeth 3 times
- Tap the tip of the tongue between the front teeth 3 times
- Gather and swallow the saliva in three separate breaths following the saliva with the Mind's eye down to the Lower Dantian.

4. Opening the Sinuses

Apply pressure with the thumb to Joining Valley or Large Intestine 4 (LI 4) located on the back of the hand at the midpoint of the second metacarpal bone along the radial border. In Chinese Medicine the Large Intestine is paired with the Lungs. Activating LI 4 strengthens the Qi of the Lungs and treats cough and asthma.

Rotate the finger pad on the Large Intestine acupoint to the left and then to the right 10 to 12 times. Then as you breathe in, apply pressure to the point. Release the pressure while exhaling. Repeat 5 to 20 times.

Apply pressure with the index fingers to Welcome Fragrance or the Large Intestine 20 (LI 20) pressure points situated lateral to the nasal passages in the nasolabial groove. Combined with LI 4 these points open the nasal passages.

Rotate the finger pads to the left and then to the right, 10 to 12 times. Then as you breathe in, apply pressure to the Large Intestine pressure point. Release the pressure while exhaling. Repeat 5 to 20 times.

Rub the sides of the nose with the sides of the index fingers. Apply pressure only on the downward beat from the mid eyebrow point to the end of the nose. Repeat 100 times with natural breathing. Palms are facing away from the body.

5. Press "Tin Dat" or Window of Sky Point

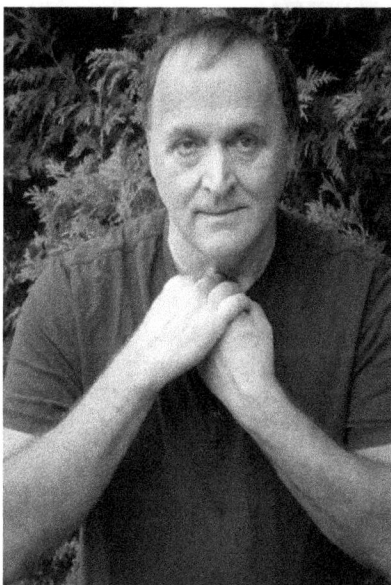

This point is good for all throat disorders and for upper chest Qi stagnation issues such as asthma and wheezing, as well as for pain and tightness in the upper chest.

- Place the 3rd finger of both hands one over the other on the CV 22 Window of the Sky Point. Inhale and open the chest moving the elbows away from the body, imagining the bright white color of the Lungs.
- Exhale lowering the elbows while putting pressure on CV 22.
- On exhalation, pronounce the healing sound for the Lungs –
See...ee...ee. Repeat 5 to 20 times.

6. Opening the Heart and Lung Meridians

Stand with the feet shoulder width apart arms resting along the sides of the body.

Inhale letting the left arm float upward to shoulder height at a 45-degree angle from the center of the body. Rotate the forearm so the thumb is pointing towards the earth. Exhale with double breath extending the arm back stretching the arm, forearm and chest, opening the Lung and Heart meridians.

Inhale as the palm returns to the front facing posture and the arm moves back to the 45-degree position. Exhale lowering the arm to the sides of the body. Repeat the same movement with the opposite hand. The movement of the arms originates in the shoulders. Repeat 6 to 12 times.

Repeat the same movement but with both hands at the same time. Repeat 6 to 12 times.

7. Activate the Great Vertebrae

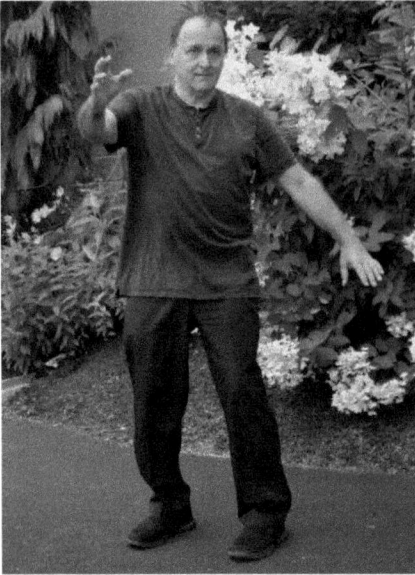

The Great Vertebrae is the meeting point of all Yang meridians of the body. It is where cold enters the body at the energetic level. It is important to keep this energy gate open to help strengthen the body's protective energy or Wei Chi.

The arms form a "T" extending away from the sides of the body at shoulder height. Move one palm forward in a circular motion to gather Qi. Turn the palm so it faces the chest area moving it towards the lungs and down to the side of the body.

The front arm gathers Qi and sweeps past the chest area cleansing the Lungs, releasing the stagnant Lung Qi deep into the earth. The spine rotates but the hips do not move. During this time, the other arm reaches back getting ready to gather Qi. Execute the same movement on the opposite side of the body. Repeat left and right 9 to 18 times in a rhythmical motion.

8. Opening Chest Center

The Chest Center, located on the sternum at the center of the chest, plays an important role in the distribution of Qi throughout the body. It unbinds the chest and helps relieve shortness of breath and the inability to speak clearly.

First open the arms to a **"T" Stance,** arms shoulder height. Extend the center of the chest forward on inhalation and release on exhalation, moving the chest center back and forth as if it were a hinge. Repeat 9 to 18 times.

Step forward with the left leg, opening the arms wide at shoulder height extending the sternum outward. Repeat the opening and closing of the chest an additional 9 to 18 times.

Bring the arms back to the sides of the body. Step to the opposite side and repeat the exercise 9 to 18 times. Keep the back leg straight and the front leg bent so that the knee tracks over the center of the foot. At the end of the repetitions return to the original standing posture.

9. Energizing Lung and Heart

On inhalation open the arms wide, expanding the chest outward. Visualize clear, fresh energy entering the Heart and Lungs.

On exhalation bring the forearms towards the chest closing the fists lightly. Imagine squeezing water out of the Lungs like you would with a damp cloth. On exhalation, pronounce the healing sound for the Lungs – **See...ee...ee.** Visualize stagnant energy moving out of the Heart and Lungs. Repeat 9 to 18 times

After the required repetitions, move the arms back to the "T" stance, open the chest wide, smile to the Universe, and drop the arms down to the sides of the body.

10. Expelling Stagnant Qi from the Lungs

Step forward with the left foot into a forward leg stance. The back leg is straight with a soft knee. The front leg is bent with the knee tracking over the center of the front foot. Lightly close the fingers in the shape of a seashell, thumb and index finger touching. This connects the Lung and Large Intestine Meridians.

Inhale, moving the palms up the front of the body. The palms are facing the body and slightly upwards. Separate the palms at mid-chest height opening the chest.

Exhale, moving the hands forward in a circular motion. The movement is executed from hip to shoulder height and is like the turning a wheel in front of the body. Repeat 6 to 9 times.

Move back to the original position. Then step forward with the right foot into a forward leg stance. Repeat the same movement 6 to 9 times on the opposite side.

On inhalation, as the palms move up the front of the body imagine you are dredging stagnant Qi from the Lungs. On exhalation as the palms extend away from the body, imagine you are sending the stagnant Qi far into the Universe.

11. Activating the Kidney Meridian

Pound the navel and lower back alternately with loosely closed fists 6 to 9 times. Continue but shift one hand to slapping the shoulder region, while the other continues to pound the lower back. Switch shoulders and repeat 6 to 9 times each.

12. Lift-Up Kidney Method

This exercise energizes the Lower Dantian. It involves Reverse Belly Breathing and the gentle lifting of the anus and perineum.

The exercise, also called Kidney Qi Gong, strengthens the Kidneys thus helping them capture the Qi from the Lungs on inhalation. Weak Kidney Qi can lead to shortness of breath. This method is also good for the excretory system, and helps prevent hemorrhoids, colon cancer and localized infection.

The Lift-Up Kidney Method helps increase sexual energy, prevent premature ejaculation, and prolapse of the anus, uterus and stomach. This method can be combined with the Microcosmic Orbit Meditation.

Feet together, heels touching, move 70% of the body weight to the front of the feet to activate the Bubbling Spring Kidney 1 point. Bring the palms to the navel, women right hand first, men left hand first.

Do not put pressure on the abdomen with the palms. The hands can also rest in any position. Inhale gently contracting the abdomen and lifting the anus. Exhale and relax, bringing the Mind to the Lower Dantian. Repeat 10 to 50 times.

On inhalation, visualize the energy moving in a circular fashion from the navel to the Hui Yin or center of the perineum to the Ming Men and back to the navel where you exhale and relax the whole body.

If a space does not move it becomes stagnant and problems can result. Movement creates energy. Reverse Belly Breathing creates a smaller space in the abdomen massaging the internal organs creating heat and energy.

The Lift Up Kidney Method is a powerful exercise that should be executed with caution. Start practicing this style with a maximum of 10 to 20 repetitions working your way up over a period of weeks to 100 repetitions. Never do more than 20 repetitions at a time without resting for a few moments.

13. Closing

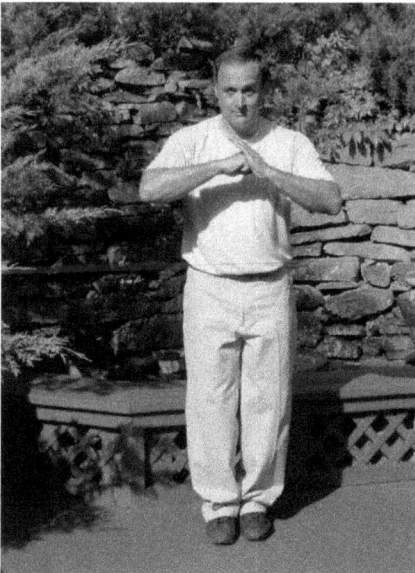

The form ends with a massage of the abdomen, face and head. The abdominal massage helps consolidate the Qi in the lower abdomen and descend rebellious Qi.

- Collect Qi by opening the arms and resting the palms over the Lower Dantian, right hand under for ladies and left hand under for men.

- Turn the hands in a spiral movement on the abdomen 9 times. Move to the left with small to big circles, then to the right with big to small circles. Keep the hands over the abdominal area.

- Bring the hands to the front of the body, palms together. Rub the palms together vigorously and, as you inhale, place them over the face, fingers pointing towards the sky.

- As you exhale, wipe the palms over the face to the sides and back of the head so the thumb and index fingers touch. Repeat 6 to 9 times.

- Bend the tips of the fingers. Inhale, and as you exhale brush back firmly with the pads of the fingers over the eyebrows, along the centerline of the head, to the back of the head 3 to 6 times.
- With the ears between the middle and index fingers, massage the sides of the head by moving the hands up and down 100 times.

- Massage the ears by pressing the thumbs along the outside of the ears against the sides of the head three times.
- Pull the ears out and then down with the thumb and the index fingers.

- Drum the Qi by placing the cupped palms over the ears with the fingers lying on the back of the head. Drum 3 sets of 9 for each of the three following methods – alternating fingers, all fingers together, snapping middle finger over ring finger.

- Drop the palms to throat level, finger pads resting below the ears on the jaw line. In a twisting motion, massage the front of the throat with the base of the palms with alternating hands. Repeat 9 times. Repeat the same movement but with both hands 9 times.

- Bring Qi down to the sides of the body and release the Qi deep into the earth. Gather Qi with the palms and place them over the abdomen, thumbs overlapping slightly at the navel, men right hand over left, and women left hand over right.

- Use the Mind to expand the body outward as big as the Universe. Inhale letting universal Qi enter the body. Exhale with the sound SOONG vibrating both the nose and whole body from head to toes. Repeat 3 to 6 times.

Qi Gong for Anxiety

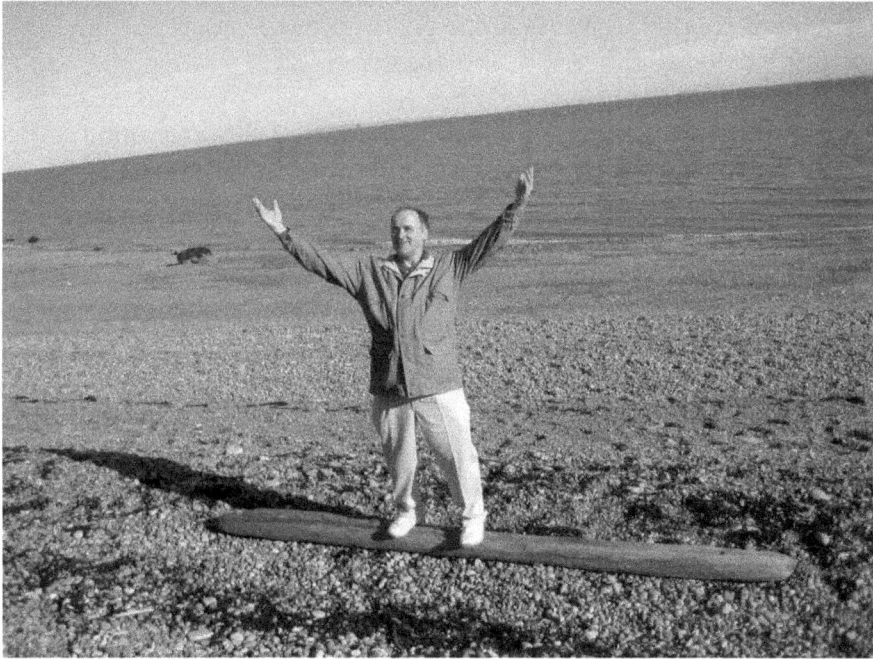

The word anxiety comes from the root word meaning "I cannot breathe" or "I'm chocking." Poor posture and shallow breathing mainly centered in the chest keeps us in a perpetual state of hypertension. The tension resulting from anxiety may over time lead to pain, disorder and disease. Inner relaxation is therefore not a luxury. It is key to health.

Qi and breath are one and the same. Qi Gong activates the breath helping reduce anxiety. Overtime the breath becomes deeper, slower, and continuous like a silk thread.

The movement of the respiratory diaphragms massage the internal organs improving digestion. The gentle movements and postures of Qi Gong open and close the body. They warm and massage internal tissue, encouraging the flow of blood, lymph, hormones and intercellular fluid. Hemoglobin levels increase as well as the production of white and red blood cells.

Blood protein levels also increase significantly, resulting in increased absorption of oxygen from the lungs and improved circulation of oxygen rich blood to the rest of the organs.

The spinal muscles elongate. Its ligaments become suppler and range of motion increases with a resulting profound effect on the nervous system fostering increased awareness and a greater sense of calmness and wellbeing.

Energetic Roots of Anxiety

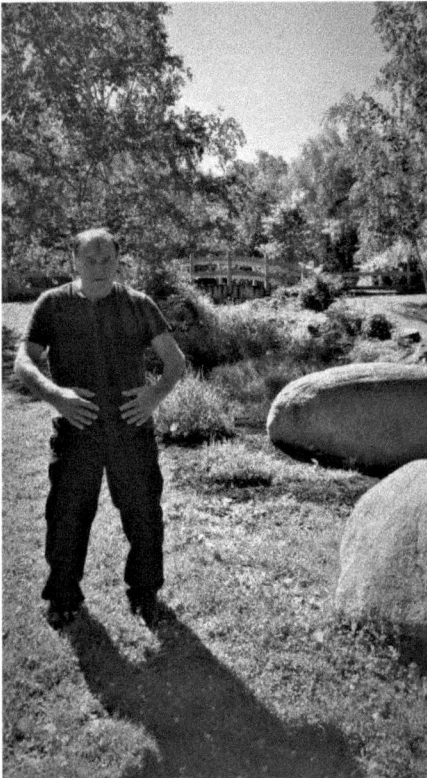

In TCM anxiety is mainly a Yin disharmony characterized by an imbalance in the fluid metabolism - blood, lymphatic fluid, hormones, intercellular fluids. A major factor in any disorder is stagnation of Qi.

This condition can over time lead to Heat rising which causes the fluids in the body to dry up. The Heat rising contributes to the feeling of anxiety and restlessness. Heat rising can turn into fire that can affect the Heart and disturb the nervous system leading to headaches and insomnia.

Qi Stagnation can also bring about an accumulation of phlegm which can cause digestive disorders such as abdominal distension and discomfort often accompanied by belching. Phlegm creates energy that is dense and sticky. The sticky energy makes the body movement feel heavy and rises to the head making the mind feel foggy.

Anxiety's exterior expression can be both Yin and Yang. It is Yin when it undermines our ability to act. It is Yang when it makes us frantic and tense. Like all energies it can shift back and forth according to conditions moving from a yin to a yang state and back again.

Gentle body movement is effective in stimulating the Qi and body fluids and, with proper diet, can help counter the effects of yin type of anxiety. Grounding exercises like standing Qi Gong can help calm the nervousness and agitation that accompanies the Yang type of anxiety.

The practice of Qi Gong has a deep, calming effect while heightening awareness. Increased awareness of what is happening around and inside of us allows one to attenuate the effects of anxiety. The mind that is anxious is the same mind that can help us work out our anxiety. Our natural mental awareness is an ally. You cannot heal what you cannot feel.

The Qi Gong approach in dealing with anxiety looks at the total field of energy – feelings, attitudes, behaviors – rather than splitting it up into separate parts. Practitioners of Qi Gong tend to breathe more deeply, resulting in increased oxygen consumption. The heart rate is slower but more powerful resulting in increased stroke volume. They are more alert but with negligible muscle tension and demonstrate improved powers of concentration, coordination and inner balance.

These are all signs of an unobstructed flow of energy that enables life to flourish. If the flow of energy is blocked, then like stagnant water, energy putrefies. Tension is what blocks the flow of Qi. Qi Gong practice relieves tension and clears blockages.

A full and more stable energy flow is less likely to be obstructed by the tensions of everyday life. A higher energy level can accommodate a wide variation of energy patterns associate with our physical, mental and emotional states. The ups and downs of anxiety and agitation do not overwhelm us.

Anxiety, worry and stress block our ability to feel what is happening in our bodies. After a little tension release our natural sensitivity to the body begins to be restored. By cultivating an imprint or pattern of what it feels like to be without tension, we can revert to this relaxation and awareness state when needed.

When we practice Qi Gong, we experience the total energetic field that lives both in and around us. The more we are open to it the more we can draw from it. Developing our sensitivity to sight, sound, smell, touch and taste provide a gateway to connecting with the constant movement of energy around us. We can ease persistent anxiety and draw the mind in any direction at any moment.

The exercises offered under the Qi Gong for Anxiety style can be combined with medical treatments or self-help methods offered by other health care professionals. You need not practice all the exercises. Start by choosing the exercises that are of benefit to you.

When practicing Qi Gong respect your body's physical and emotional limits. Do what is good for you. Practice no hurray, no worry, and smile from the Heart.

Qi Gong for Anxiety 13-Style Form

The following Qi Gong form calms the Mind, nourishes the Heart and strengthens the body. It helps you let go of the harmful emotions and negative thoughts that nourish the anxiety. For better results, in addition to the practice of Qi Gong, it is also necessary to reduce stress in daily life and nurture a positive attitude.

Spend 20 minutes outside in the early morning or early evening every day without wearing glasses or contacts. There can be clouds. The natural light strengthens the pineal, pituitary and hyper thalamus glands. This activity helps regulate serotonin, melatonin and dopamine hormones which govern general mood.

Enjoying more intense physical activity is helpful as it regulates the Liver which governs excessive emotions such as anger towards oneself that may lead to depression. When going for a walk, relax and let the arms swing back and forth naturally. Practice the following Qi Gong style outdoors every day if possible.

Be patient as it may take some time to see an improvement in your condition. Like in all health care systems there is no guarantee of success. Focus on the journey and not the destination.

Be Happy, No Hurry, No Worry and Smile from the Heart.

1. Relaxed Belly Breathing

Adopt a standing posture with the following indications:

- Feet shoulder width apart, 70% of body weight on the heels, knees straight but soft, abdomen pressed gently against the lower back, and chin moving in and up gently lifting the Adam's apple.

- Arms hang down the sides of the body with the palms of the hands open and facing the sides of the body.

- Anus is closed gently and the tip of the tongue is placed on the upper palate behind the front teeth.

- Practice with soft eyes that are fully open, or half closed looking towards the horizon, and *Smile from the Heart.*

- Let the body move front to back and back to front for a few moments in a spontaneous movement to let go of ingrained tension.

- Still the body and quiet the Mind. Inhale and exhale through the nose. The breath is thin, even, silent, deep and long. Inhale expanding the abdomen outward in all directions, exhale letting the chest drop down towards the hips.

Do not force the inhalation. Inhale 70% of capacity, and exhale 100% of capacity. Be aware of the quiet space between exhalation and inhalation. Let the inhalation rise on its own from this quiet space. Practice 30 breaths or for 5 minutes.

2. Awareness Meditation

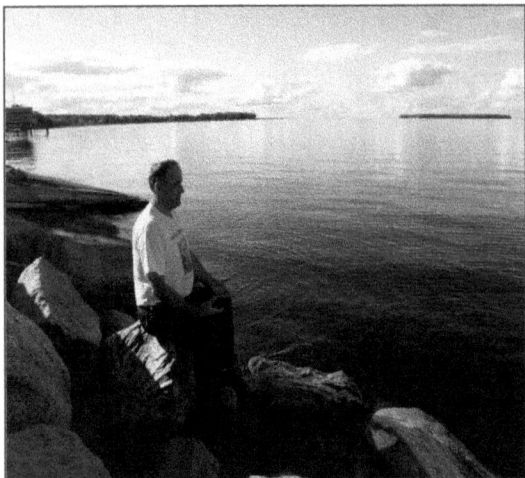

Practice awareness meditation standing, sitting or lying down before and after sleep, after walking, when you feel stressed or anxious, or at the end of a Yoga or Qi Gong class.

When standing the arms hang down the sides of the body. The body weight is 70% on the heels. Drop the tailbone down. The crown of the head is suspended from above.

When sitting, the back is straight, chin in, body relaxed, and the palms are facing up resting on the upper thighs or facing down if you suffer from high blood pressure.

When meditating on your back, the head is slightly elevated on a four-inch pillow. Hands are at the sides of the body, palms facing you.

As you inhale become aware of any movement in the body: pain, discomfort, thoughts, sensations, emotions, sounds, images. Stay non-attached like an objective observer of your internal landscape. As you exhale let the distractions that catch your attention flow down deep into the earth.

In the presence of an ailment such as an ache or pain that has a specific and definite location, you can meditate on that area to facilitate healing. This brings Qi to the affected area. As you inhale, look within the affected area with an attitude of non-attachment. Exhale relaxing the area. As you exhale allow any uncomfortable sensations to disappear.

124

Then using the Mind, direct Qi to the area. If there is heat or agitation imagine a cooling or reducing effect. If there is cold or weakness imagine a strengthening or warming effect. If there is stagnation imagine an opening and refreshing effect. Continue for 5 to 10 minutes. Practice Relaxed Belly Breathing throughout this form.

3. Coming Up for Air

Adopt a standing posture:

- Feet shoulder width apart, 70% of body weight on the heels, knees straight but soft, abdomen pressed gently against the lower back, and chin moving in and up gently lifting the Adam's apple.

- Arms hang down the sides of the body with the palms of the hands open and facing the sides of the body.

Coming Up for Air disrupts the anxiety pattern and helps you experience a different sense of time and space. Transform how you feel when sitting, standing or walking. Use the Mind to open the body to the Universe.

Relax in a standing posture for a few minutes. Inhale with Relaxed Belly Breathing opening the palms slightly and expanding the chest outward.

Smile from the Heart. Exhale and relax. When standing on inhalation move 70% of the body weight forward to the balls of the feet. On exhalation move 70% of the body weight back to the heels. Repeat 6 to 12 times.

This exercise can also be done with a rotation of the cervical spine to one side on inhalation looking slightly upward to where the ceiling meets the wall, moving back to center on exhalation. Repeat left and right for 6 to 12 times.

Opening the body to the Universe allows powerful universal Qi to enter the body. A simple smile calms the body's nervous system and bathes the internal organs with a nectar-like substance.

4. Connecting Palm Center to the Three Dantians

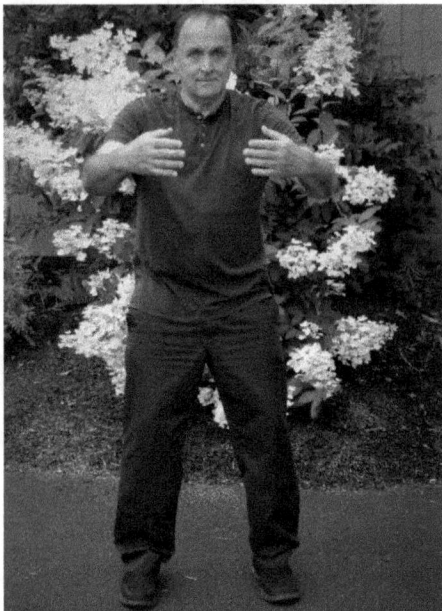

This exercise helps activate the three Dantians. Hold the palms about two fist widths away from the Lower Dantian. The palms are relaxed, rounded like seashells with fingers parallel to the floor.

Using the Mind, connect the palm center to the Lower Dantian via the Sea of Qi or Qi Hai energy gate located about two to three finger widths below the navel. Inhale with Relaxed Belly Breathing expanding the palms outward to gather Qi from the Universe. Exhale extending Qi into the Lower Dantian via the palm center. Repeat 6 to 12 times.

Raise the arms to mid-chest height, palms facing the center of the chest. Using the Mind, connect the palm center to the Middle Dantian via the Chest Center or Dan Zhong energy gate. Inhale with Relaxed Belly Breathing expanding the palms outward to gather Qi from the Universe and exhale extending Qi into the Middle Dantian via the palm center. Repeat 6 to 12 times.

Raise the arms to shoulder height, palms facing the forehead. Relax the eyebrows. Using the Mind, connect the palm center to the Upper Dantian via the Yin Tang or mid-eyebrow energy gate. Inhale with Relaxed Belly Breathing expanding the palms outward, gathering Qi from the Universe.

Exhale, moving the palms slightly forward sending Qi from the palm center into the brain cavity activating the pineal gland. Repeat 6 to 12 times.

Then on inhalation arch back reaching up with the palms towards the sky embracing the Universe. Straighten the torso with the palms facing the top of the head and let universal Qi pore over the body.

Flex and extend the knees creating an up and down movement of the palms activating the flow of Qi in and out of the Crown Point. before lowering the arms down the front of the body palms facing the earth.

Reconnect with the Lower Dantian and repeat the complete sequence 3 to 6 times.

5. Arm Swinging to Strengthen Kidney Qi

Strong Kidney energy is required to be able to move forward in life. This exercise helps strengthen the Kidney energy while releasing stagnation in the Kidney meridians.

The arms feel open and light, hanging down the sides of the body. Rotate the hips gently back and forth. The arms will swing with the movement of the hips. Relax the hips and lower back gradually increasing the amplitude of swinging. Repeat for a few minutes.

Then fists lightly closed, gently tap the abdomen just below the navel with one hand while the other hand gently taps the sacrum on the back of the body. Repeat for 30 times alternating hands.

Then add a palm slap to the chest area just above the breast with one hand while the other closed fist simultaneously taps the sacrum. Alternate the tapping of the abdomen/sacrum with the chest slap/sacrum tap. Repeat 12 times before switching to the other side of the chest and repeat another 12 times.

6. Spinal Wave

The Spinal Wave is practiced with Reverse Belly Breathing. It massages the internal organs and opens the spine where the Governing Vessel is located connecting the Kidneys with the Heart and the Brain.

Place the left palm over the area just below the navel and the right palm over the center of the chest. Inhale contracting the lower abdomen, gently raising the anus. The center of the chest will naturally extend forward. Exhale and relax. Repeat from 10 to 30 times. This is a very powerful exercise. Be gentle to avoid injuring the internal organs.

Once you are comfortable with this exercise on inhalation imagine fire moving up the back and on exhalation imagine water flowing down the front of the body.

7. Tapping Abdomen to Release Emotional Trauma

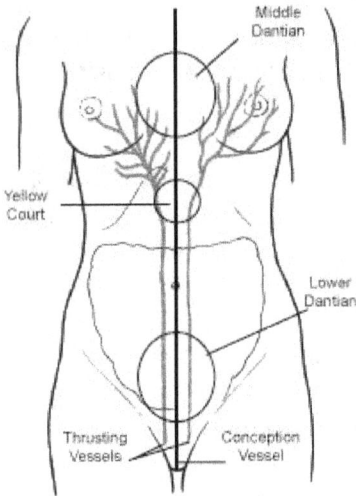

Deep rooted emotional trauma often stagnates in the tissues of the gut. This exercise helps release this long-standing tension helping you return to a more normal energetic and emotional state.

Place the left hand over the Heart at the ST 16 or Breast Window just above the nipple and the right hand over the center of the abdomen four fingers width above the navel at REN 13 or Upper Cavity.

Rub the center of the abdomen from side to side with the palm of the right hand to warm an relax the area. Then join the finger and thumb pads of the right hand together and tap the area vigorously for about 30 to 60 times or until the tension subsides.

Rest the right palm on the abdomen. Bring the finger pads of the left hand together. Tap the area just above the left nipple 30 to 60 times.

Repeat the sequence 3 times alternating from the tapping of the center of the abdomen and the tapping of the Breast Window.

Rest the palms of the hands comfortably left hand over the Heart and right hand over the center of the abdomen. After practicing Relaxed Belly Breathing for a few moments let the left hand slide off the upper abdomen.

Extend the palm towards the ground releasing stagnant Qi deep into the center of the earth. Repeat the same movement with the opposite hand alternating hands clearing out stagnation in the Yellow Court or area just below the sternum. The trunk rotates with the movement of the hands. Repeat 10 to 20 times.

The Breast Window point helps release chest fullness and pain. In the context of this exercise, its proximity to the Heart may be factor in helping connect the Heart energy with the emotions hidden in the gut or Yellow Court.

The Yellow Court is located inside the body near the center of the abdomen. In ancient China citizens requesting an audience with the Emperor would be required to wait in the Yellow Court until the Emperor was ready to acknowledge their presence.

In Chinese medicine the Heart represents the Emperor. This exercise helps release deep rooted emotions lodged in the Yellow Court, so they can be acknowledged by the Emperor Heart.

8. Raising Hands to Expel Toxic Emotions

The arms are resting along the sides of the body. On inhalation raise the hands up the front of the body with the palms facing slightly up and towards you. Be aware of any troubling emotions that may be contributing to your anxiety.

At chest height separate the hands wider than shoulder width opening the chest. The elbows are heavy. Rotate the palms so they face away from the body.

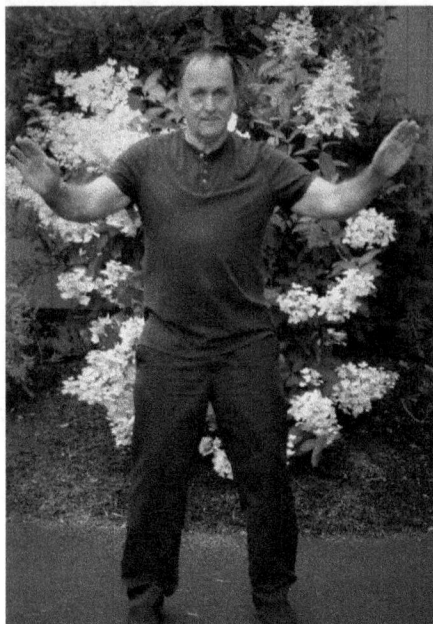

On exhalation push the palms away from the body at a 45-degree angle, sending hurtful emotions and negative thoughts far into the Universe. At full arm extension, relax the hands releasing tension in the palms before bringing them back in and up the center line of the body. Repeat 6 to 12 times.

Repeat the same exercise raising the hands higher so the palms face the forehead before they rotate outward and extend away from the body on exhalation. Repeat 6 to 12 times.

Then with palms facing each other raise the hands up the center line of the body towards the sky. On maximum extension separate the hands while rotating the palms outward.

Lower the hands to the sides of the body and repeat the exercise 6 to 9 times. Inhale as the palms move up the center line of the body and exhale as the palms extend outward towards the sides of the body. Practice Relaxed Belly Breathing throughout this form.

9. Harmonize the Kidneys and the Heart

According to the Five Element Theory the Kidneys represent the Water element and the Heart represents the Fire element. The Kidney Water helps cool or regulate the Heart Fire and the Heart Fire helps heat up the Kidney Water.

Each organ system depends on the other to help maintain a state of balance. The following exercise helps regulate the connection between these two organ systems.

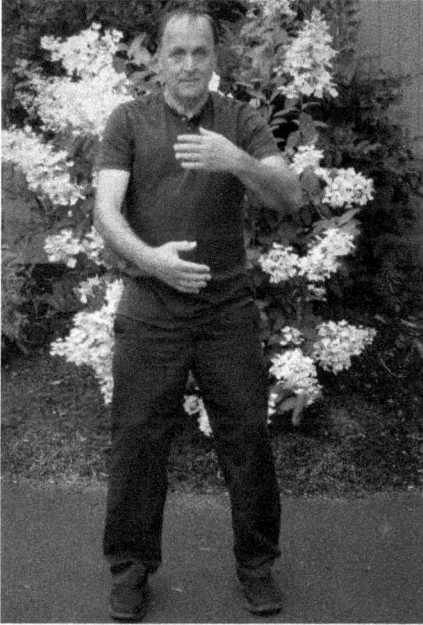

Place the left hand above the Heart with the palm facing the chest, about a fist width away from the body. Place the right hand at the level of the navel with the palm facing the lower abdomen about a fist width away from the body.

Breathe naturally for a few minutes, letting the Mind focus on the Heart Fire. The Heart is warm and red in color. Then continue breathing for a few minutes letting the Mind focus on the Kidney Water. The Kidneys are cool and a dark midnight blue color.

Then switch hand positions. For a few minutes focus on warming the Kidney Water with the Heart Fire. Then focus on cooling the Heart Fire with the Kidney Water. Switch hands and start again. Repeat 6 to 9 times.

With the hands back at the starting position, left hand above the Heart, right hand above the lower abdomen, focus on normalizing the Heart Fire and Kidney Water.

10. Angle Breathing

Place the thumb, index and ring finger pads of the right hand on the Bai Hui or Crown Point of the head, with pads of the fingers gently touching. Place the thumb, index and ring finger pads of the left hand about three fist widths away from the Mid Eyebrow Point or Yin Tang.

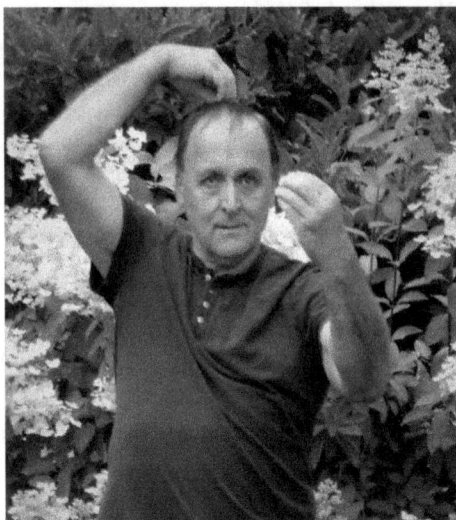

Inhale Universal energy via the Yin Tang into the brain cavity moving the left finger pads towards the forehead to gently touch the Yin Tang energy gate. Breathe out the Bai Hui energy gate far into the distance moving the right finger pads away from the crown of the head. Visualize toxic Qi releasing from the brain cavity.

Then inhale clear Qi through the Bai Hui into the brain cavity moving the pads of the right thumb, index and ring fingers back to the Crown Point. Exhale toxic Qi out of the brain cavity via the Yin Tang far into the Universe while moving the left finger pads about three fist widths away from the forehead. Repeat 9 to 36 times.

Once you are familiar with this method drop the arms to the sides of the body and use the Mind to move the Qi in and out of the acupoints without touching them with the finger pads. Repeat 9 to 36 times. Practice Relaxed Belly Breathing throughout this form.

11. Three Line Method to Relax Body

Stand with arms hanging down the sides of the body. Inhale universal energy via the Bai Hui or Crown Point of the head into the center of the body down to the Lower Dantian. Exhale Qi out the Bai Hui down the front of the body to the toes. Repeat 3 to 6 times.

Inhale universal energy via the Bai Hui into the center of the body down to the Lower Dantian. Exhale Qi out the Bai Hui down the sides of body to the outside of the feet. Repeat 3 to 6 times.

Inhale universal energy via the Bai Hui into the center of the body down to the Lower Dantian. Exhale Qi out the Bai Hui down the back, buttocks and the back of the legs to the heels. Repeat 3 to 6 times.

Then inhale universal energy via the Bai Hui into the center of the body down to the Lower Dantian. Exhale Qi out the Bai Hui down the front, sides and back of the body to the feet. Repeat 3 to 6 times. Practice Relaxed Belly Breathing throughout this form.

12. Natural Walking Qi Gong

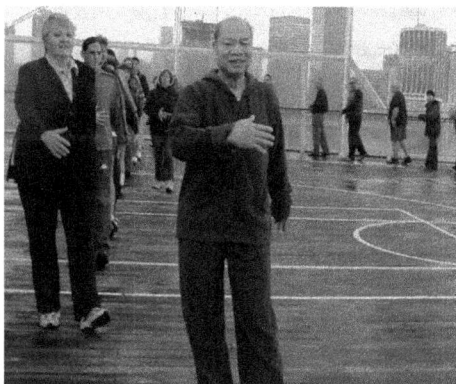

It is better to practice natural walking Qi Gong in a clean natural environment. As you walk, move from heel to ball of feet pulling the body forward with the front foot once it fully connects with the floor or ground.

Open the Ming Men or Gate of Fire located on the lower back by curling the tail bone under as if sitting on a chair. Imagine the crown of the head is suspended from above. Look far to the horizon. The body is relaxed.
The arms swing naturally back and forth along the sides of the body. The opposite leg and arm move at the same time.

Once the walk becomes natural, practice every day during regular activities with a *Smile in your Heart.*

Breathe naturally and walk like you are young with the Spirit up.

13. Harmonizing the Three Dantians
Rest one palm over the other with the tips of the thumbs touching in front of the lower abdomen. Women place the right hand on top, men left hand on top.

Inhale releasing the top hand swinging it out and away from the body until it reaches the top of the head in line with the center of the body. The thumb points towards the body and the palm faces to the side.

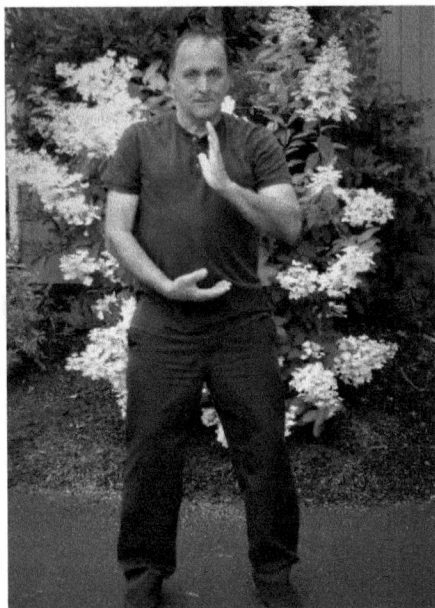

Exhale slowly dropping the palm down the center line of the body until it regains its original position in front of the lower abdomen. Repeat the movement with the opposite hand. Continue left and right for 6 to 9 times.

Then as you drop the hand down pause in front of the Yin Tang or mid-eyebrow point. Imagine the point is open like a cylinder reaching into the center of the brain. Follow the breath with your Mind in and out of the point 3 to 6 times.

Repeat the same exercise at the mid-chest point or Dan Zhong. Then with the palms in their original resting position in front of the lower abdomen, repeat the same exercise at the Sea of Qi or Qi Hai point.

Repeat with the opposite hand. Redo the exercise until the points feel open and refreshed. Practice Relaxed Belly Breathing throughout this form.

14. Closing with Self Massage and SOONG

The form ends with a massage of the abdomen, face and head. The abdominal massage helps consolidate the Qi in the lower abdomen and descend rebellious Qi.

- Collect Qi by opening the arms and resting the palms over the Lower Dantian, right hand under for ladies and left hand under for men.

- Turn the hands in a spiral movement on the abdomen 9 times. Counter clockwise: from small to big circles . Clockwise: from big to small circles.

- Place the overlapped palms on the base of the sternum and rub down the center of the abdomen to the pubic bone 6 to 9 times.

- Place both hands on the floating ribs and rub down to the pubic bone 6 to 9 times.

- Bring the hands to the front of the body, palms together. Rub the palms together vigorously and, as you inhale, place them over the face, fingers pointing towards the sky.

- As you exhale, wipe the palms over the face to the sides and back of the head so the thumb and index fingers touch. Repeat 6 to 9 times.

- Bend the tips of the fingers. Inhale, and as you exhale brush back firmly raking the head with the tips of the fingers from the forehead, along the centerline of the head, to the back of the head 6 to 9 times.

- With the ears between the middle and index fingers, massage the sides of the head with the finger pads by moving the hands up and down 100 times.

- Massage the ears by pressing the thumbs on the outside of the ears towards the head three times.

- Drum the Qi by placing the cupped palms over the ears fingers lying on the back of the head. Drum 3 sets of 9 for each of the three following methods - alternating fingers, all fingers together, snapping middle finger over ring finger.

- Drop the palms to throat level, with the fingers resting below the ears on the jaw line. In a twisting motion, massage the front of the throat with the base of the palms with alternating hands. Repeat 9 times. Repeat the same movement but with both hands moving together 9 times.

- Bring the palms down to the sides of the body and release the Qi deep into the earth.

- Gather Qi with the palms and place them over the abdomen, thumbs overlapping slightly at the navel, men right hand over left, and women left hand over right. Rest the Mind in the center of the abdomen for a moment.

- Use the Mind to expand the body outward as big as the Universe. Inhale aware of the universal Qi entering the body. Exhale with the healing sound SOONG vibrating the whole body from head to toes. Repeat 6 to 9 times.

Embracing the Void

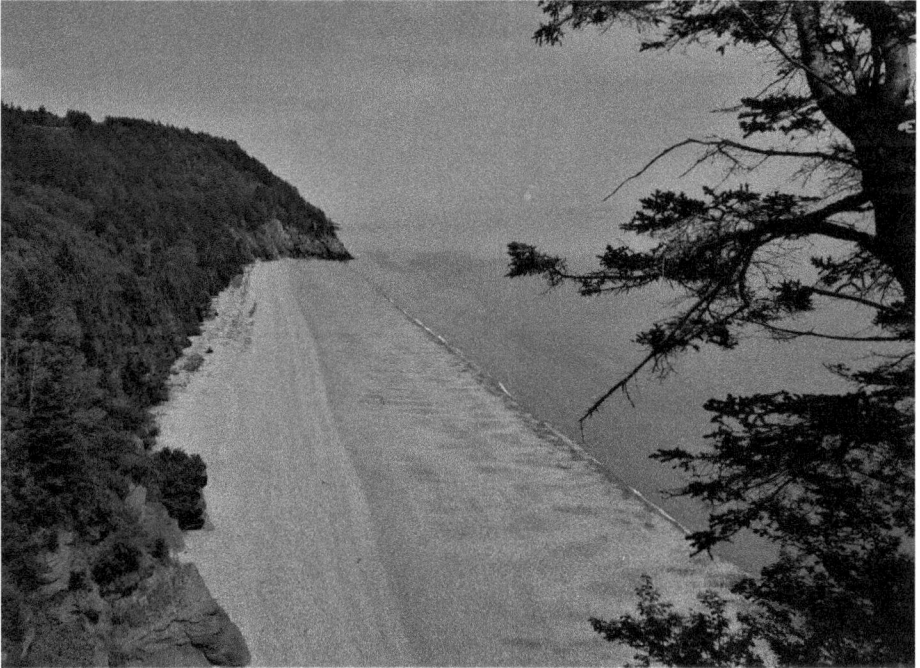

Qi Gong works with patterns of energy in and around the body. Like many forms of energy, human energy and its movements are invisible to most of us. We experience its effects. A person's energy field connects with the energy that surrounds them. Emotions constantly arise within the energy field like weather patterns.

Some energies are denser and others more ethereal. They arise from our own field of energy or from the energetic field of the Universe. A single thought can cause our hearts to skip a beat. A single breath of air can open our Minds.

In the Taoist tradition the human body is understood to be a small galaxy. Qi Gong connects our personal galaxy with the rest of the Universe, with the immense energy of the incalculable number of galaxies that surround us. Qi Gong allows us to train our own energy field strengthening our sensitivity to and connection with the vast energy field in which we live.

Imagine you are like a vast ocean of unknown depths home to inconceivable life forms capable of accepting, absorbing and purifying whatever enters it. Mental states of distress, despair and being overwhelmed respond instinctively to warmth, expansiveness and a widened horizon of awareness. A healthy relationship with our own energy and the natural energy of the Universe provides a path to human empowerment.

We act as magnets for the energy that surrounds us. Constant streams of energy come to us and pass through us. The energy of the cosmos tends to be more variable and unstable. It is associated with creativity. The energy of the earth tends to be more constant and stable and is associated with power. Qi Gong allows us to harmonize these two forces.

The mind is a renewable resource. Its power is its freshness. We can tap into that freshness – instantly. That is what our senses are constantly inviting us to do.

Dark Matter is a mysterious substance that scientists believe accounts for approximately 90 percent of the mass of the Universe. Dark Matter is invisible to the human eye, but its presence can be detected in part from its gravitational effects on visible matter.

Qi Gong science talks about similar phenomena called Void Energy. The Universe is bigger than our collective imaginations. It stretches beyond our ability to comprehend.

Like other natural phenomena, the Universe and its omnipresent Void Energy is mirrored in our everyday lives. It can be found in the pause between inhalation and exhalation, at the crest of a wave and in the space between the notes of a song. It is the turning point that creates definition and rhythm, akin to stillness in action. It gives meaning to life and animates all life.

In the hustle and bustle of everyday life we take little time to connect to our true selves, to find the eye of the storm. Those who do connect find a greater purpose in life. They can step back and see the forest for the trees.

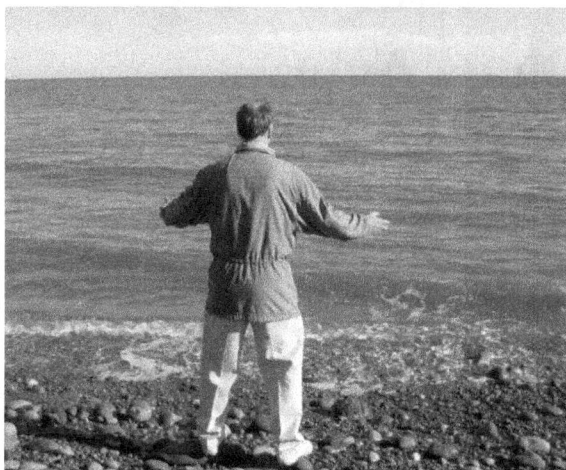

In the normal evolution of persons, Jing Qi (Essence of Body) is transformed into Qi (Energy), Qi into Shen (Spirit), Shen into Wuji (Emptiness), and Wuji into the Dao of Divinity (Origin of All).

This transformation is facilitated by the practice of stillness, breath and heart-felt awareness. Stillness relaxes the body and the Mind, breath harmonizes the Qi, and the absence of expectations brings peace to the Heart.

People who experience the void in their meditative practice become extremely relaxed, flexible and soft. Their energy is light, abundant and free flowing.

Clear away your thoughts. Open your Heart and embrace the world around you. Return to the Void, to your energetic roots. Develop a state of transparency with no Mind and no form.

In this manner, we can all enrich our present existence with the wisdom of the ages and help create a new Qi Gong Science for the benefit of present and future generations.

To further your knowledge of Qi Gong, consult my other books entitled Qi Gong's Five Golden Keys, which explores the five keys to opening the Qi door, and Dance of the Dragon - Healing Oneself & Others, which offers methods to strengthen and express healing Qi.

Authors' Note

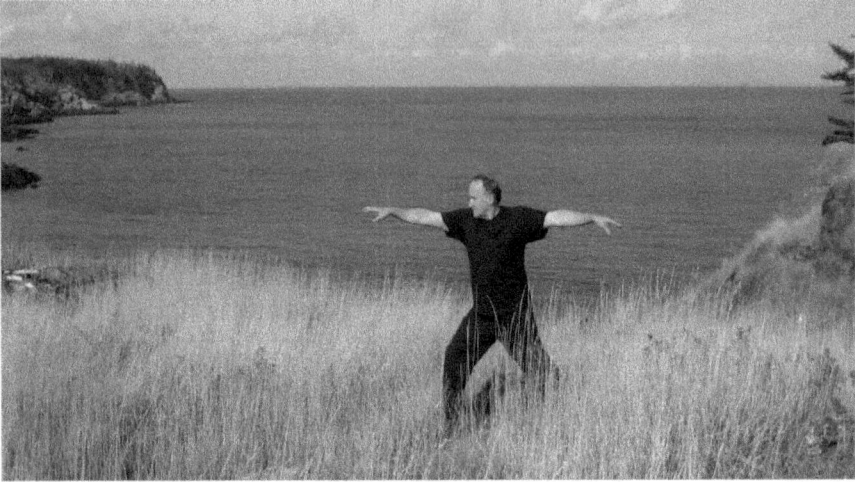

Qi Gong is a very powerful healing art. Nevertheless, benefits from practicing Qi Gong vary from person to person. For the best results, follow a healthy diet and lifestyle. Persons suffering from mental illness or epilepsy should not practice Qi Gong.

The author of this book is not a Medical Doctor. If you have any doubt about your ability to practice Qi Gong, please consult with your physician before undergoing training. This book is not intended to replace personalized medical care or treatment.

Practice One Mind Instead of Many

Stay Grounded with the Spirit Up

Smile from the Heart

References

A Brief History of Qi - Zhang Yu Huan & Ken Rose - Paradigm Publications, 2001

A Manual of Acupuncture - Peter Deadman & Mazin Al-Khafaji - Journal of Chinese Medicine Publications, 2007

Acid-Alkaline Diet for Optimal Health - Christopher Vasey, N.D. - Healing Arts Press, 1999

Anatomy of the Spirit - Caroline Myss, Three Rivers Press, New York, '96

Acupressure's Potent Points - Michael Reed Gach – Bantam Books, 1990

Chinese Medical Qi Gong Therapy - Dr. Jerry Alan Johnson - International Institute of Qi Gong, 2000

Chinese Medical Qigong Therapy - Grand Master Tzu Kuo Shih, OMD, L.Ac., and Melanie Shih, OMD, L.Ac. - Second Military Medical University Press, 2010

Chinese Medical Qi Gong - Tianjun Liu, O.M.D. & Kevin Chen, Ph.D. - Singing Dragon 2010

Dream Healer - Adam, Penguin Canada, 2003

Foundations of Chinese Medicine - Giovanni Maciocia, Elsevier, 2005

Healing Touch, A Guidebook for Practitioners - Dorothea Hover-Kramer, Delmar Tomson Learning, 2002

Life More Abundant - Xiaoguang Jin & Joseph Marcello - Buy Books on the Web.Com, 1999

Living Pain Free with Acupressure - Dr. Devi S. Nambudripad, 1997

The Chinese Art of Healing with Energy - Qi Gong Therapy - Dr. Tsu Kuo Shih, Station Hill Press, 1994

The Art of Peace - Moreihei Ueshiba, Shambhala, 1992

The pH Miracle, Balance Your Diet, Reclaim Your Health - Robert O. Young and Shelley Redford Young, Wellness Central, 2003

Wudang Qigong - Yuzeng Liu - International Wudang Internal Martial Arts Research Association, 1999

Healing with Whole Foods: Asian Traditions and Modern Nutrition - Paul Pitchford, North Atlantic Books, 2002

The Qi Gong Workbook for Anxiety - Master Kam Chuen Lam, 2014

yinyanghouse.com; taoism.about.com; biofieldglobal.org pacificcollege.edu; seventreasureshealingarts.com; lotusrootacupuncture.com; sarahjgeorge.wordpress.com longwhitecloudqigong.com; baharna.com/chant/six_healing.htm

Editor: Louise Gosselin **Photos & Revision of Texts:** Louise Gosselin, Maurice Lavigne and FreeDigitalPhotos.net.

Diagrams: Microcosmic Orbit - Wikimedia by Bostjan46; Chakra - Flickr by Tania_b33; Mu/Shu Points by Oxford University Press.

For more information or to book a Qi Gong workshop contact the Fredericton Wellness Clinic Inc

Email: WClinic@Outlook.com
Tel: 506-452-9795
Web: WClinic.ca
Facebook: facebook.com/FrederictonWellnessFitness

Copyright: Fredericton Wellness Clinic Inc
Fredericton, NB, CANADA June 2017
ISBN 978-0-9949347-6-5